W9-BKF-920

3 1668 07110 3151

PRAISE FOR THOMAS W. PHELAN

What parents are saying:

"This book **changed our lives**."

"My three-year-old has become a different little girl, **and she is so much happier now**."

"**The ideas in this book work!** It really is like magic! I feel like **I am back in charge**."

"Simple, clear, concise, and **easy to follow**."

"**I highly recommend this book** if you need a method of dealing with your little one(s) that keeps everyone calm."

"Extremely **helpful and informative**."

"A **great book** for any parent!"

"**I was desperate for a change** in my family dynamics. **This book was the answer!**"

"**Fantastic book** that really helps with toddler tantrums. **My husband and I both read it** and now **we are disciplining in the same way**. This book has been a **lifesaver!**"

"*1-2-3 Magic* **simplifies everything** I've read in other books, which makes it **very easy to follow**. Our home has become **a much more positive place**."

"**Easy to read** and easy to follow."

"**Buy this book; read this book; follow the instructions in this book!** I highly recommend this to anyone involved in disciplining children."

"*1-2-3 Magic* **made parenting fun again**."

"All I have to say is that **the ideas in this book WORK!** It really is like magic!"

"**This book is amazing!** My three-year-old was having major tantrums 4–6 times a day, screaming at the top of his lungs. After applying 1-2-3 Magic, he rarely has meltdowns."

"*1-2-3 Magic* **takes the stress out of discipline**."

"**It's such a relief to not feel like I'm constantly yelling at someone!** If you want to see a fast improvement in your child's behavior, check out *1-2-3 Magic*."

"Fantastic book that **really helps with my toddler's tantrums**."

"This is the **one-stop, go-to book** that we have referred to time and again."

"This book is a great tool! It **helped me feel confident and proud of my parenting skills**."

"The methods are described clearly and they are **easy for any parent to follow**. I am **already seeing an improvement** in the way I react to my five- and seven-year-olds."

"We feel **more in charge** and **in control**."

"**Saved my blood pressure** and my relationship with my kids."

"**This book isn't just about time-outs and discipline**; it encompasses an entire parenting philosophy."

"**I highly recommend this book** to any parent who is s**pending more time yelling at or nagging** their children **than smiling at and laughing with them**."

"**Thank you**, Dr. Phelan, for **sharing the results of your extensive research** and experimentation with the rest of the world!"

"*1-2-3 Magic* **saved my marriage**."

"This is a **must-read** for all parents."

"Our little girl had gotten full-blown into the terrible twos and **I was desperate to get the calm back in my household**. She caught on to this method in one day. **Our house is a pleasant place to be again**."

"This book **really helps!**"

"If you have challenges with your kids and you consistently follow the directions in this book, **you will have such a better relationship with your children**."

"I have read many discipline books and tried many different methods. **This was the one that worked for our family**."

"Thank you, Dr. Phelan! **You are a lifesaver!**"

What experts are saying:

"**This book is easy to read and navigate**. As an in-home therapist I need lots of parent-friendly tools to use with families, and this is one of them. **I highly recommend it!**"

"As a parent and a school social worker, I highly recommend this book/system to everyone."

"**A wonderful book to use with parents in therapy** to assist with parenting skills."

"As a school guidance counselor, **I highly recommend this book** to both parents and teachers."

"Great book! **I am a pediatrician and I recommend it to my patients**."

"**I've recommended this book for years** in my practice as a psychotherapist."

"**This is a staple** in my child therapy practice's pantry of goods."

"As a pediatrician, **I believe all caretakers should read** *1-2-3 Magic* and I cannot recommend it highly enough."

"As a mental health professional, I've found *1-2-3 Magic* to be **the most powerful method** of managing kids aged 2-12 that I've ever come across."

All About
ADHD

A Family Resource for Helping Your Child
SUCCEED WITH ADHD

THOMAS W. PHELAN, PhD

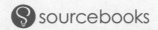

Copyright © 2017 by ParentMagic, Inc.
Cover and internal design © 2017 by Sourcebooks, Inc.
Cover design by Erin Seaward-Hiatt
Cover images/illustrations © Rob & Julia Campbell/Stocksy

Sourcebooks and the colophon are registered trademarks of Sourcebooks, Inc.

All rights reserved. No part of this book may be reproduced in any form or by any electronic or mechanical means including information storage and retrieval systems—except in the case of brief quotations embodied in critical articles or reviews—without permission in writing from its publisher, Sourcebooks, Inc.

This publication is designed to provide accurate and authoritative information in regard to the subject matter covered. It is sold with the understanding that the publisher is not engaged in rendering legal, accounting, or other professional service. If legal advice or other expert assistance is required, the services of a competent professional person should be sought.—*From a Declaration of Principles Jointly Adopted by a Committee of the American Bar Association and a Committee of Publishers and Associations*

This book is not intended as a substitute for medical advice from a qualified physician. The intent of this book is to provide accurate general information in regard to the subject matter covered. If medical advice or other expert help is needed, the services of an appropriate medical professional should be sought.

Published by Sourcebooks, Inc.
P.O. Box 4410, Naperville, Illinois 60567–4410
(630) 961–3900
Fax: (630) 961–2168
www.sourcebooks.com

Originally published as *All About Attention Deficit Disorder* in 1996 by ParentMagic, Inc.

Library of Congress Cataloging-in-Publication Data
Names: Phelan, Thomas W., author.
Title: All about ADHD : a family resource for helping your child succeed with
    ADHD/ Thomas W. Phelan, PhD.
Description: Naperville, Illinois : Sourcebooks, [2017] | Includes
    bibliographical references and index.
Identifiers: LCCN 2016053260 | (pbk. : alk. paper)
Subjects: LCSH: Attention-deficit hyperactivity disorder--Treatment. |
    Attention-deficit-disordered youth--Treatment. |
    Attention-deficit-disordered children--Treatment.
Classification: LCC RJ506.H9 P524 2017 | DDC 618.92/8589--dc23 LC record
available at https://lccn.loc.gov/2016053260

Printed and bound in the United States of America.
VP 10 9 8 7 6 5 4 3 2 1

CONTENTS

INTRODUCTION

ATTENTION-DEFICIT/HYPERACTIVITY DISORDER (ADHD) IS
a chronic condition in which core symptoms of excessive inattentiveness, impulsivity, and hyperactivity cause significant impairments in a
person's school, work, social, and home life. ADHD is a challenge for
families, schools, and society for a number of reasons.

The prevalence of ADHD in children in the United States averages
between 5 percent and 7 percent, while in adults, the prevalence is
about 3 to 5 percent.[1] Most of the time, ADHD does not go away, and
lifelong management is therefore necessary. ADHD has been found
in countries and regions worldwide, although its prevalence varies
depending on geographical location.[2] ADHD is complicated—it does
not usually come by itself. More than two thirds of children and adults
with ADHD also have a second (comorbid) psychiatric disorder, and
many have a third.[3] These comorbid problems commonly include
oppositional defiant disorder, conduct disorder, substance use disorders, anxiety, and depression. Individuals with ADHD are also more
prone to learning disability and motor incoordination.[4]

ADHD strongly impacts families, and ADHD runs in families.
About half of all mothers with children diagnosed with ADHD have
experienced clinical depression. Parents with children with ADHD
are more likely to experience marital conflict, separation, and divorce.
Siblings of children with ADHD often feel mistreated and neglected,
and they themselves are also at higher risk for ADHD as well as other

problems. Because ADHD has a strong genetic component, it is very common for families to have several children and adults with ADHD living under the same roof.[5]

The prevalence, complexity, and negative impact of ADHD are the bad news. The good news is that reliable, useful, and scientifically accurate information about ADHD has become more and more widespread. More and more, children with ADHD are being properly diagnosed and treated. More classroom teachers are being trained to understand and manage ADHD, producing corresponding benefits to children with the disorder, their classmates, and to the teachers themselves. Fewer parents these days, as opposed to a decade or more ago when less was known about the disorder, believe the myth that they somehow caused ADHD in their children due to bad parenting or argue about "which one messed up this kid." ADHD is now understood as a neurological, genetic, and treatable condition, not an indication of failings within the family. Many parents of children with ADHD and many adults with ADHD greet the diagnosis with some relief. They are glad to learn the problem has a name, that it is "not their fault," that mental health experts know a lot about this condition, and that a course of management/treatment can be defined.

Further benefits have come from the recognition that most kids with ADHD do not outgrow their symptoms, which has led to diagnosis and effective treatment for many adults as well as to useful accommodations for college students with the disorder and affected employees in the workplace.

A diagnosis, however, is not magic, and it is only the beginning of the usually lifelong process of dealing with the symptoms of ADHD. *The most important part of the treatment process is education about ADHD.* That's what this book is about. You may be a parent trying to deal with your child's first-grade teacher, discussing medication for your son with a pediatrician, attempting to explain the disorder to the grandparents, or trying to manage your own periodic depression. Or you may be an adult with ADHD trying to handle a difficult job, get along with your girlfriend, or keep track of your money.

Whatever the case, you want good knowledge about ADHD

to help you raise your child or to run your own life as an adult. Dependable facts are emotional gold. You need to understand basic symptoms, how these symptoms affect school, home, workplace, and peer relations, what it's like to grow up with ADHD, what causes ADHD and the genetic aspect of the problem, how to predict the future (prognosis), how ADHD is diagnosed, what treatments are useful, and what treatments (though often highly touted!) are useless.

Unfortunately, information about ADHD on the Internet is too often simply distorted and idle chatter. Stories about ADHD in the media are too often sensationalized and negative, although this problem seems to be lessening. I hope *All About ADHD* will provide you with the latest reliable and scientific evidence about this disorder—in a simple, readable format—so that you can maximize your happiness and the happiness of those you love.

All About ADHD is based on my own personal experience as a parent, grandparent, and clinical psychologist who has worked with children and adults with ADHD for over forty years. ADHD will always have a personal, family side as well as a clinical, scientific side. In my opinion, to really grasp the problem and deal effectively with it, you need to understand both.

1

THREE VIEWS OF ADHD

IN THIS CHAPTER, WE'LL examine ADHD from three points of view: (1) ADHD according to the *DSM-5*, (2) what it's like to actually have or live with ADHD, and (3) ADHD viewed as fundamentally a problem of self-control.

The *DSM-5* Criteria for ADHD

The American Psychiatric Association's *Diagnostic and Statistical Manual of Mental Disorders (DSM)*, now in its fifth edition, defines attention-deficit/hyperactivity disorder. The *DSM-5* is used by physicians, mental health professionals, and insurance companies for diagnosis and treatment recommendations. According to the *DSM-5*, several criteria must be met for an individual to qualify as having ADHD. Basically, the person must show a pattern of inattention and/or hyperactivity-impulsivity that fits the following criteria:[1]

1. Persistence: symptoms have lasted for at least six months.
2. Number of symptoms: persistence of six or more symptoms for children through sixteen-year-olds; five or more symptoms for age seventeen and up.

3. Early onset: several symptoms existed (not necessarily diagnosed) prior to age twelve.
4. Frequency and severity: symptoms must be inconsistent with developmental level and not just a result of oppositional behavior or inability to understand tasks or instructions.
5. Clear evidence of impairment: the ADHD symptoms must significantly interfere with or reduce a person's ability to function.
6. Symptoms occur in two or more settings: symptoms must be present in multiple contexts, such as school, work (for adults), home, and social situations.
7. Symptoms not due to another mental disorder: ADHD symptoms do not only occur during a psychotic disorder and cannot be explained by another mental disorder, such as a mood disorder, anxiety disorder, substance use, and so on.

The *DSM-5* classifies symptoms according to inattention, hyperactivity, and impulsivity.[2] For the sake of simplicity, the abbreviated description of each item is below. The first list includes manifestations of *inattention*:

a. fails to pay close attention to details; makes careless mistakes
b. has difficulty following instructions and completing tasks
c. has difficulty sustaining attention in work or play and is easily distracted
d. often fails to listen when spoken to directly
e. has difficulty organizing tasks and activities
f. avoids tasks requiring sustained mental effort
g. often loses things
h. often distracted by extraneous stimuli
i. is forgetful in everyday tasks

The second list includes symptoms associated with *hyperactivity* or excessive motor activity, and impulsivity, acting without thinking:

j.   fidgets or squirms in seat

k.   leaves seat when remaining seated is expected

l.   runs about or climbs in situations where such activity is inappropriate

m.   has difficulty playing quietly

n.   acts as if "driven by a motor"; always going

o.   talks excessively

p.   blurts out answers before questions are completed

q.   has difficulty waiting their turn

r.   interrupts or intrudes on others

Here's how the diagnosis is made: if a child qualifies for six or more items on both lists, the diagnosis is attention-deficit/hyperactivity disorder, combined presentation (ADHD-C). Individuals with this diagnosis have trouble paying attention, and they are also overly active and/or impulsive. If a child qualifies for six of the nine inattentive items but does not meet six of the nine hyperactivity/impulsivity criteria, he or she would be described as having attention-deficit/hyperactivity disorder, predominantly inattentive presentation (ADHD-PI). These children are not restless or disruptive, but they do have trouble focusing on tasks, sustaining attention, and organizing and finishing things.

Finally, what if you meet the hyperactivity/impulsivity criteria (six or more items) but not the inattentive criteria? The *DSM-5* does recognize a predominantly hyperactive-impulsive presentation (ADHD-PHI), but there is some controversy about whether or not ADHD-PHI is truly a separate entity. The opinion of many experts is that the predominantly hyperactive-impulsive presentation is really a younger version of the combined disorder.

The *DSM-5* also makes a couple of other changes in ADHD criteria. Unlike the previous edition, the *DSM-IV*, the manual describes ADHD "presentations" instead of types, recognizing the fact that the different kinds of ADHD are not really rigid "types" but more like fluid conditions that may change with time. In addition, the number of items required to qualify for one of the two scales (inattentive and hyperactive/impulsive) was lowered for adults from six to five. This change was made because many adults can still experience ADHD impairment even though they may not hit the six-item cutoff.

Over the years, there has been controversy over whether the condition sluggish cognitive tempo (SCT) is a subtype of ADHD or a distinct disorder.[3] Although it does not yet appear in the *DSM-5*, characteristics of SCT include daydreaming, slow processing speed, or sluggishness.[4] These are characteristics that resemble ADHD, predominantly inattentive. SCT is not thought of as a deficit in overall intelligence. Most research on SCT to date involves children, but the feeling is that this is a new clinical entity separate from ADHD.[5]

Living with ADHD

The *DSM-5* provides an accurate but still largely clinical view of ADHD. Symptom lists are a useful and necessary part of diagnosis, and the *DSM* criteria have been researched and standardized extensively. But symptom lists do not describe what it is like to be—or to live with—a child or adult with ADHD. Below are eight characteristics that are often experienced by individuals with ADHD. These real-life descriptions will give a better picture of how ADHD affects not only a person's life, but also the lives of their family and friends.

Our list, of course, includes the core ADHD symptoms: inattention, impulsivity, and hyperactivity. But we'll provide a fresh perspective by adding five new entries. Children and adults who qualify for ADHD-C will often show all of the attributes on our list. On the other hand, people with ADHD-PI may fit only items 1, 6, and 8.

1. inattention (distractibility)
2. impulsivity
3. hyperactivity
4. difficulty delaying gratification
5. emotional overarousal
6. noncompliance
7. social problems
8. disorganization

Inattention (Distractibility)

The child with ADHD has an attention span that is too short for his age. He cannot sustain attention on a task or activity, especially if he sees that activity as boring or semi-boring. Naturally, most children with ADHD spend a good deal of their time in school, and we hear from them over and over again how "boring" it is. Ask children with ADHD what they don't like about school, and they may simply say, "the work." It is a significant strain for these children to try to stay on task; they are fighting an invisible problem they don't understand. The stress they experience is considerable and, for those who have not gone through it themselves, hard to imagine. As they get older, children with ADHD often begin to feel like they are stupid, and they are often accused of being lazy—experiences that will likely damage their self-esteem.

What sometimes confuses the picture, however, is that many children with ADHD *can* pay attention (or sit still) for limited periods of time. I have found they may be able to do this when they are in situations that have one or more of four particular characteristics. These characteristics are:

a.　novelty
b.　high interest value
c.　intimidation
d.　one-on-one with an adult

This temporary ability of children with ADHD to sit still and concentrate can amaze people who have previously only seen these kids in their hyperactive mode. It can also produce plenty of missed diagnoses! Examples of these special situations? The first two weeks of a school year (novelty), watching TV or playing video games (high interest value), a visit to a pediatrician's office (intimidation), going to a ball game alone with Mom or Dad (one-on-one), and psychological testing (all four!).

Another way of looking at the attention problem is to think of it as distractibility: the ease with which the child can be taken off task by some other stimulus. Children with ADHD respond automatically to anything new. Many children with ADHD can tell you how much it bothers them when the garbage truck pulls up in the parking lot during social studies, when someone's using the pencil sharpener, or when they have their socks on inside out.

In my experience, distractors for individuals with ADHD come in four forms: visual, auditory, somatic, and fantasy. Visual distractors are things within the child's field of vision that draw his attention away from his work or task. For example, someone walks by and causes him to look up, and then he may not be able to return to his work. Auditory distractors are things the child hears that bug him. They can be obvious, loud noises or quieter sounds like the ticking of a clock, someone tapping a pencil on a desk, or another child sniffing. These things may not seem bothersome to you, but they are to children with ADHD.

Somatic distractors are bodily sensations that take away the child's attention. I have seen a number of children who can hardly stand it when the seam in their sock is not in the right place. They become very fidgety and can't concentrate. The same results occur if their stomach is growling, if their chair is uncomfortable, or if they have a headache.

> **Key Concept**
>
> Distractors come in four forms: visual, auditory, somatic, and fantasy.

Fantasy distractors are thoughts or images going through the child's mind that have more appeal than schoolwork. We all daydream, but children with ADHD are often identified by teachers as excessive daydreamers. The child might start thinking of his new video game, or lunch, or—if he's old enough—about a girl.

Some children may be more vulnerable to certain kinds of distractors than others. Some kids, for example, complain more about things that they hear than things that they see. That's why it helps with the diagnosis if a child can describe in his own words what kinds of things get him off task.

What is the biggest distractor for children with ADHD? Very likely human conversation. When children with ADHD say they can't concentrate when other children talk around them, this is probably not an excuse; it's a very real problem.

Impulsivity

The second trait on our list is impulsivity: acting without thinking or doing whatever happens to come to mind without regard for the consequences that may follow. Impulsive acts by children with ADHD can range from trivial to extremely dangerous.

In the extremely dangerous category is impulsive behavior that threatens the life of the child with ADHD or the life of others. For example, one boy I worked with started playing with matches in a wastebasket in his living room. The flames intrigued him, but they soon reached up to the curtains and then spread. No one was hurt, but the house was lost. Another five-year-old patient of mine with ADHD almost drowned when he went to a pool with his father. The father turned away for only a short time, but the child saw the water, saw other kids jumping in, and thought "fun." His thought processes didn't extend as far as remembering that he didn't know how to swim. He was pulled off the bottom of the pool several minutes later. Fortunately, he was still alive.

Other impulsive ADHD behavior is more along the lines of less damaging mischief. In school situations, teachers will often recognize children with ADHD by their tendency to blurt things out in class and forgetting to raise their hand. Other times, children will blurt out something intended to be funny or smart-alecky. Many children with ADHD attempt to be the class clown, and some of them are quite clever and really *are* funny. This type of behavior, however, presents the teacher with a major class management problem as the whole group of kids gets off track.

Impulsivity can also seriously impair the social interactions of children with ADHD. When frustrated, they may yell at other children and sometimes even physically strike out or push others around in an attempt to get their way. Their impatience about having to immediately be the first in line and their tendency to grab other children's things can be constant sources of irritation to others.

Some people say that children with ADHD have a "stop, look, and listen" problem.[6] In other words, when entering a new situation, they don't take the time to stop, look at what is going on, listen to what is being said, and then respond appropriately. Children with ADHD tend to do whatever comes naturally—or automatically.

Children with ADHD do not have a well-developed ability to either visualize consequences or to talk to themselves about what is likely to result from some of their actions. Some children who impulsively steal, for example, just look at the money lying on their parents' dresser and think, "Wow! Neat!" So they take it. It may occur to them later that their father will almost certainly miss the five dollars that was sitting on top of the dresser earlier in the day, but by then, the damage has been done.

Children with ADHD often lie for the same reason. When asked if their homework is done, the child with ADHD may quickly respond yes because they don't want the potential hassle of having to do their homework *now*, and they don't think of what will happen later when they are caught. Parents are often amazed and mystified by this phenomenon. They can't imagine anyone being so "stupid" as to lie—not just once, but repeatedly—"knowing" he will certainly be caught later.

Hyperactivity

Hyperactivity is a probable symptom of ADHD, especially in younger, preadolescent children. Hyperactivity involves gross-motor restlessness, not just being fidgety. Parents describe their children as being always on the go or acting like they are "driven by a motor." Being around this constant activity can be draining and irritating for parents. Repeated—but useless— suggestions to "Sit still!" or "Calm down!" may often be heard around the house.

> **Key Concept**
> Hyperactivity means gross-motor restlessness, not just being fidgety.

Even among children who are hyperactive, the hyperactivity will usually greatly diminish by adolescence.[7] This explains why people used to think that hyperactivity would be outgrown. The typical reduction in activity level with age doesn't mean, however, that restlessness and other ADHD symptoms are gone; these characteristics usually continue into adulthood.

In addition, hyperactivity itself is *not* constant. Children with ADHD, combined presentation type, can sometimes sit still in situations that are new, fascinating, somewhat scary, or one-on-one.

Girls with ADHD tend to be less hyperactive (and less impulsive) than boys with ADHD. But not all children with ADHD are hyperactive, as evidenced by the existence of ADHD, predominantly inattentive. This diagnosis is meant for children who have difficulty concentrating but who do not present a lot of behavioral problems. These children do exist, but among children with ADHD, they are in the minority. Children with ADHD, predominantly inattentive, often fall through the cracks in a school system, because they don't aggravate anyone very much. Because disruptive behavior drives school referrals, the children with the most severe cases of ADHD tend to be the ones who receive the most aggressive treatment.

Difficulty Delaying Gratification

Another trait I have commonly found in children with ADHD is difficulty delaying gratification. You might think of this one as simply a bad case of *impatience*. To parents, it often feels like the child is saying, "I want what I want when I want it, and I want it now! If you don't give it to me, I'll have a temper tantrum, or I'll badger you until you give it to me!"

When children with ADHD get an idea in their heads about something they want, they can be remarkably persistent in pursuing it. This kind of behavior often makes shopping with them a miserable experience. Unless you're at a store that has nothing of interest to them, they will see a million things and want all of them in sequence. This difficulty in delaying gratification makes some parents feel defeated before they even leave home, because they think just about any shopping trip is going to mean buying the child something. Parents may begin to avoid going to the store with their children so they don't have to deal with the embarrassment of horrible public tantrums when they refuse to buy their children something they want.

At school, difficulty handling delays can manifest itself in a number of ways. Children with ADHD may shove others in order to be first in line or run down the hall bumping into people to be the first one out for recess. In schoolwork, impatience can show itself in hurried, messy work. Children with ADHD simply want to get it out of the way as soon as possible, rather than take the time to do a good job on it. This attitude can mean not reading directions and doing a lot of schoolwork the wrong way.

Difficulty with delay can also result in sloppy handwriting. However, since many children with ADHD also have trouble with fine motor skills, it is sometimes hard to tell if they are rushing, if their sloppy work is the result of a problem with fine visual-motor coordination, or if it is some combination of both.

The tendency toward impatience can also mean any holidays that involve gifts—such as birthdays, Hanukkah, or Christmas—can be stressful. Children want their presents early, or they get overly excited and badger their parents incessantly.

Some children with ADHD have trouble with soiling or wetting themselves because of their difficulty with delay. They are out playing and having a good time, they feel the need to go to the bathroom, but they *can't put off the next few minutes of play*. The urge to go to the bathroom builds, they keep repressing it, and then—in a moment of physical exertion—they lose control and soil or wet themselves. Even after this happens, some children will continue to play, because they still don't want to go in.

If you think of this kind of mentality, you can easily imagine why one of the words that frequently comes out of the mouths of children with ADHD is "Boring!" Imagine you are always thinking about what the next exciting thing to come along is going to be. In the meantime, you feel like you are just sitting around, and the minutes are crawling by. Things would seem pretty boring to you too.

Emotional Overarousal

Another quality that often accompanies ADHD is an extreme intensity of feelings and emotions.[8] Children with ADHD also make sure those around them are aware of their emotional state. I have been saying for years that emotional overarousal is not mentioned on the

DSM-5 lists, but it probably should be (and it probably will be in future *DSMs*!).

Perhaps the two most common emotions involved in this regard are happiness or excitement on the positive side, and anger on the negative side.

Happy children with ADHD are frequently overly excited. They get into what I call a "hyper silly" routine, especially in unstructured groups with other children. They may run around frantically, talk loud, and act goofy. Parents may be embarrassed by this display, and other children may find such behavior unusual.

Who doesn't know what's happening? Children with ADHD. They are often notoriously insensitive to social cues. They don't notice the displeased expression on someone's face, pick up on a negative tone of voice, or even hear the words spoken. As many parents know, one of the least effective adult tactics in these situations is to plead or yell "Calm down!" That suggestion is like throwing gasoline on a fire. Usually, it helps if the child can be gently removed from the situation for a while in order to regain control.

When angry, on the other hand, children with ADHD can erupt into horrible temper tantrums. These tantrums sometimes appear like rages well beyond the degree of frustration most people would express. Because of moments like these, some parents wonder if their children are psychotic. However, the rage may subside as quickly as it started, and then the child may be off to some pleasant, new encounter.

Although emotional overarousal with ADHD is often thought of in terms of these two extremes—excitement and anger—research now shows that other emotions, such as anxiety and sadness, can be exaggerated as well.[9] By the time they are teens, for example, perhaps 30 percent of children with ADHD may also meet *DSM* criteria for an anxiety disorder. Another 20 percent may meet criteria for depression.[10] These psychological problems all involve, to varying degrees, the exaggeration of certain negative emotions.

Some children with ADHD, for example, experience extreme separation anxiety. They have a hard time leaving their home or parents. Others experience sadness and, in older children, depression.

Fortunately, these periods of depression or sadness typically do not last as long in the younger children, as mood changes are typical in children with ADHD.

What about guilt? Children with ADHD probably have fleeting moments of guilt, but—according to many parents—this is not one of the emotions they tend to feel too intensely. Internalizing problems like these are more common with ADHD-PI. Of course, many parents of youngsters with ADHD-C wish their kids felt more guilt! In fact, these parents often worry that their child doesn't have a conscience.

Noncompliance

Many children with ADHD, especially those with ADHD-C, have a hard time following rules, and they often present significant discipline problems. This prompts some adults to think they have to do a better job of teaching these children the rules. Yet actually knowing the rules is not the problem. During quieter times, children with ADHD may not only be able to remember the rules, but they may also be able to recite them. However, in the heat of battle, they tend to forget them and how to apply them. Emotional overarousal, hyperactivity, and impulsivity take over. ADHD is not a problem of knowing what to do; it's a problem with these children actually *doing* what they already know. Performance, rather than knowledge, is the issue.

Some ADHD noncompliance involves aggressive behavior. Such children are often pushy with other children and can be intolerant of the needs of their siblings. They can create a lot of domestic turmoil. Parents are often torn between their desire to treat their children fairly and equally and their knowledge that the child with ADHD often starts many (not all) of the fights around the house. Other aggressive, noncompliant behavior includes arguing and yelling.

Noncompliance is the reason that 50 to 60 percent of kids with ADHD also qualify for a *DSM* diagnosis of oppositional defiant disorder (ODD).[11] Children with ODD (at younger ages, mostly boys, and often children with ADHD-C) are negative, defiant, hostile, and argumentative. These kids lose their tempers easily, seem to have a chip on their shoulders, like to annoy others, and blame everyone else for whatever goes wrong.

As you can imagine, younger children who have ADHD and ODD are more likely to be diagnosed with conduct disorder (CD) as teenagers.[12] Teenagers with CD have advanced to nastier, much more noncompliant, and much more dangerous kinds of behavior. Teenagers with CD violate age-appropriate norms. For example, they often smoke, drink, use illegal drugs, and engage in sex at early ages. Children with CD have impaired conscience development, and they may physically hurt others, steal, vandalize property, or even torture animals. Many of them will turn out to have antisocial personalities as adults.[13]

Recent research has pointed out some disturbing but potentially useful information: the transition from younger kids with ADHD/ODD to older kids with CD is often aggravated by greater social adversity and more psychopathology in families.[14] Parents who are inconsistent disciplinarians, for example, and parents who suffer from depression, substance abuse, and ADHD themselves often increase the chances of their kids running into trouble as teens and adults. In other words, as a parent, you don't cause ADHD, but you can certainly make it worse.

What about instances of passive noncompliance, such as forget-fulness, losing things, and distractibility? Noncompliance can be not particularly harmful to anyone other than the passively noncompliant person herself. This is especially true when ADHD-PI is involved. Because of their inattentiveness, general disorganization, and forgetful-ness, children with ADHD-PI (and perhaps SCT as well) don't clean their rooms, forget to feed the dog, and don't do their homework. A motto of one of our many ADHD parent support groups is this: "Don't ever ask a child with ADHD to do three things in a row." Sometimes, it is hard enough to get children with ADHD to finish just one task. You're lucky if she finishes one! A parent may ask a child to take out the garbage. She agrees, which may be unusual in itself, and heads off to get it. On the way, however, she passes the TV. That's it—the garbage is forgotten.

Social Problems

For too many children who have ADHD, peer problems are a big part of their lives. I have often felt that children with ADHD-C will often be *rejected*, while children with ADHD-PI will be *overlooked*. The result is often heartbreaking for the child's parents.

Competitiveness is often based on similarity, and many children with ADHD-C have a difficult time getting along with other children, especially those who are the same age and sex. The child's interpersonal problems usually come from being too intense, bossy, aggressive, and competitive. Children with ADHD-C suffer from what is often referred to as low frustration tolerance (LFT). Most of these children hate losing, and they may resort to cheating, fighting, or changing the rules in the middle of a game in order to get their way.

One fascinating study asked this question: "How long does it take for a person to create a lasting negative impression?" The study was conducted with children with ADHD at a summer camp, and the answer to the question was three hours! It only took three hours to establish a bad reputation that lasted for the whole summer.[15] How can children so rapidly guarantee their reputation as difficult? The answer to this question was simple: aggressive behavior. Push, bite, bully, hit, and generally be loud and obnoxious.

Aggressive behavior from children with ADHD often results in two outcomes: (1) isolation, and (2) playing with children several years younger. The reasons for the isolation are obvious. But why do children with ADHD play with younger children? We'll explain that in chapter 2.

Unfortunately, interpersonal problems are very difficult to change, especially the bad reputation of a rejected child. Research has pointed out that even when kids do change their behavior, their bad reputations stay put.[16] This reality is especially discouraging, because one of the strongest predictors of adult success in life is one's social skills.[17] Making matters worse is the fact that social skills training for ADHD-C doesn't work very well—at least in the manner in which it's been done so far.[18]

On the other hand, some children with ADHD-PI get along just fine with playmates. Often, these children are very easygoing, pleasant, and somewhat passive—the opposite of the often "in your face" type of child with ADHD-C.

Disorganization

If you had all the seven of the ADHD characteristics mentioned so far, you would probably have trouble with organization too. Children and adults with ADHD are often disoriented and forgetful; they lose track of time, and they frequently lose things.

Children with ADHD are often *amazingly* forgetful. What drives many parents crazy is when children do their homework and then lose it before they even get a chance to turn it in! Where did it go? It's on the floor in the backseat of the car or perhaps under the bed. Many times, the homework actually does get to school in the child's folder. But it may have been a math paper that was stuck in a social studies folder, so it wasn't found until three weeks later.

> **Key Concept**
> Kids with ADHD are often disoriented and forgetful; they lose track of time, and they frequently lose things.

There seems to be a psychological law that dictates that trouble concentrating leads consistently to forgetfulness. Kids with ADHD often forget what they studied last night for a test the next day. They often lose their schoolbooks, their clothes, their cell phone, and even their toys. One nine-year-old boy came into my office one day and mentioned he had played a Little League game the day before. When asked the score, the boy said, "It was 17 to 2." When asked who won, he said he didn't remember! People without ADHD usually vividly recall a win or loss by such a wide margin.

Children with ADHD may also have a poor sense of time and place. They can never seem to get home on time, even if they have a watch or a cell phone. Some of this disorientation, of course, is due to the problem of delaying gratification—children with ADHD don't want to leave what they're doing to go home. But they also just don't pay much attention to time. This trait is painfully obvious in the morning when the entire family is trying to get out the door. I have found that early morning ADHD-induced chaos is one of parents' biggest complaints; everyone leaves the house stressed and starts the day in a bad mood.

Family members may also find that the child with ADHD is always borrowing their things, and then losing them. Fathers might go through many sets of tools before a child with ADHD grows up and leaves home. Alternatively, I have found that some children with ADHD are "prowlers" and "hoarders." They seem to be constantly snooping around the house, and they may actually steal other people's things with no intention of giving them back.

As mentioned earlier, children with ADHD-C will likely fit all eight of the characteristics just mentioned. Those who are diagnosed with the ADHD-PI variety, however, will show only inattention, noncompliance (more the passive rather than the defiant kind), and disorganization. ADHD-C is often noticeable and diagnosable as early as age three. What stands out at these very young ages is not inattention but disruptive behavior. Preschool children with ADHD are obvious primarily because of impulsivity, impatience, emotional overarousal, hyperactivity, noncompliance, and social aggressiveness that is excessive for their age.

Kids with ADHD-PI, on the other hand, don't usually face significant challenges until they hit school, where their daydreaming, forgetfulness, and inability to finish projects become more of a problem. Even in the early grades, however, these children are often overlooked because they cause little or no trouble.

ADHD and Self-Control

So far, we've examined the *DSM-5* symptom lists, and we've also taken a detailed look at what it's like to have ADHD or live with someone who has ADHD. Another way of looking at the ADHD concept is the idea that attention-deficit/hyperactivity disorder is fundamentally a difficulty with one's ability to self-regulate or self-control. Proposed by Dr. Russell Barkley in *ADHD and the Nature of Self-Control*, this point of view suggests that the basic problem is one of "behavioral disinhibition." Barkley's theory has been well accepted by researchers in the field, and it has triggered a lot of interest in and research on what is often referred to as executive functioning, the ability to self-regulate in the interest of long-term goals.

Barkley's theory is based on a concept called *behavioral disinhibition*. Children with ADHD have trouble *not* responding to the newest, most interesting, most predominant, or most fascinating stimulus that comes along, especially when *they should be doing something else*. If you are taking a casual stroll through the forest, for example, it's OK to bend down to examine a bug, watch a hawk soaring high above, or even wander off the path to follow a green leopard frog. If you are sitting in a classroom taking an ACT test, however, it's not OK to daydream about your boyfriend or girlfriend, watch a squawking crow flying by the window, or become so irritated by your neighbor's sniffling that you walk out of the room. (This has happened!)

Barkley proposes that people with ADHD have trouble holding back and waiting before prematurely making some kind of internal or external response. As mentioned earlier, this is a kind of "stop, look, and listen" problem. Barkley takes the idea further, however. Because the individuals with ADHD respond impulsively, Barkley says, they do not take the time or get a chance to use the four executive functions that are the essence of self-regulation.

The four executive functions include working memory (holding relevant facts in your mind), internal speech (talking to yourself), emotional regulation (calming down or motivating yourself), and reconstitution (creating a useful solution or response).[19] In other words, the executive functions involve the ability to calm down and think things over—even if it's only for a second or two. People with ADHD not only do not use these executive functions well in the first place, they also do not get a chance to practice and hone their executive skills over the years, because they're too often reacting too quickly.

For example, take two high school sophomores living in Chicago. Noah has ADHD-C; Mark does not have ADHD. Both are finishing their supper at about 6:00 p.m. on a dark, cold Tuesday night in

February. Both boys are enthusiastic basketball fans, and they want to watch an important Bulls game on at 7:30 that evening. Noah's and Mark's parents remind them they have to get their homework done before they can watch the game. The boys head to their bedrooms to get started (a minor miracle in itself).

At 7:15, Mark is nearly done with his algebra assignment—the last of his homework for the evening. Noah is on his computer, playing his favorite fighter pilot game. His homework is untouched.

What happened? Let's do a slow-motion replay of each boy's mental processing during the minutes right after dinner. Noah, who has ADHD, went up to his room. He sat down at his desk and opened up one of his school folders, but his first reaction upon looking at his first homework assignment was a strong emotional revulsion toward doing his homework at all. He then glanced at his computer, thought about the fighter pilot game, and started playing. What he did was an automatic, impulsive response more than a real decision. The game was fun—a lot more fun than homework.

Mark also went up to his room intending to do his homework, *also* felt revulsion at the idea when he sat down, and—like Noah—also glanced at his computer and thought about the entertaining fighter pilot game. But then he stopped (behavioral or response inhibition) and thought a little bit. He remembered (working memory) that he had algebra, Spanish, and a lot of history to do—and there was a Bulls game on at 7:30. *I really want to watch that game tonight, and the only way my parents will let me is if I finish my homework*, he thought to himself (internal speech). While controlling his distaste for the unpleasant task of doing homework (emotional regulation—calming down), he recalled that the last time he had not done his algebra homework, he had wound up embarrassed in front of the whole class. *I don't want that to happen again!* he thought (emotional regulation—motivation). He also really wanted to watch that Bulls game. Getting his homework done before the game would be his reward (motivation) for getting his work done.

The difference between the two boys is clear. You can see that ADHD involves a difficulty in being constructively oriented toward the future and engaging in goal-directed activity. As Ned Hallowell, a child and adult psychiatrist who specializes in ADHD and is the coauthor of the book *Driven to Distraction*, said, "When [you have] ADHD, there are only two kinds of time: now and not now. I have a final exam next week. Not now!"[20]

So perhaps the name for ADHD should really be "BID: behavioral inhibition disorder," and there should be a greater focus on impulsivity (behavioral disinhibition), rather than on hyperactivity (hyperkinetic reaction of childhood) and inattentiveness (attention deficit disorder), which have taken center stage for years.

> **Key Concept**
> ADHD involves a difficulty in being constructively oriented toward the future and engaging in goal-directed activity.

2

HOME, SCHOOL, AND FRIENDS

THIS CHAPTER WILL EXAMINE how ADHD traits can affect a child in the settings of school, home, and social situations. We'll focus primarily on children (chapters 15–17 will focus more on adults), and we'll examine the effects of two kinds of ADHD:

a. ADHD-combined presentation (ADHD-C)
b. ADHD-predominantly inattentive presentation (ADHD-PI)

As was discussed on pages 5–6, we are taking the point of view that ADHD predominantly hyperactive/impulsive presentation (ADHD-PHI) is really the same as ADHD-C. Also, until more research is available, we'll consider sluggish cognitive tempo (SCT) to be a part of the ADHD-PI category.

School: ADHD-C

If you were asked to create an environment that could drive a child with ADHD crazy on a daily basis, you probably couldn't come up with anything worse than school. School requires that the child not only sit still but also concentrate on material that he often finds uninteresting. *Boring* is one of the most commonly words used by children with ADHD to describe school.

Because of his difficulty with rules and self-control, a child with ADHD-C is often a significant negative force in the classroom. He will stand out like a sore thumb, and all the other children will be aware of who he is and how much trouble he gets into. He will often fall into a vicious cycle with his teacher: he acts up, she tries to control him, he resists by acting up more, she attempts to exert more control, and on and on. By April, the hostilities can be extreme, and by that time, the parents are also likely to be involved in the confusion.

Even though the IQ of children with ADHD-C can be the same as or better than their classmates, their academic performance can be uneven. Teachers may notice them excessively daydreaming when they are distracted by internal stimuli. At other times, they may blurt out answers without raising a hand or clown around by making jokes or silly noises.

Most children with ADHD want to do well just as much as other kids do, and they can have spurts when they indeed do well. But because they are continually bumping their heads against an invisible concentration and motivational problem, these kids will not be able to sustain their effort. Some children with ADHD can have an entire year where they are able do fairly well and improve their behavior and learning. When this occurs, it is usually due to a very positive teacher interaction effect. Brenda, for example, gets Mr. Smith in the third grade. He likes Brenda, and he is willing to put up with a certain amount of goofing off. Brenda also likes Mr. Smith and is willing to work for him more than she usually does. The year goes fairly well, and Brenda's parents start to think she is "maturing."

Then fourth grade rolls around, and Brenda gets Mrs. Hammond. Mrs. Hammond thinks ADHD is a fabricated diagnosis and says she "doesn't believe in it." She doesn't particularly like Brenda, and she thinks her parents make too many excuses for her. Brenda reciprocates her teacher's negative feelings toward her, and in a short period of time, Brenda's behavioral problems start up again.

What do we know about the IQs of children with ADHD? In my experience, kids with ADHD are about as smart as anyone else. Some are quite bright, most are average, and some are of below-average intelligence. Regardless of their IQ, children with ADHD often struggle with using their intelligence effectively because of their problems with paying attention and sitting still.

With regard to learning disabilities, it's a different story. These kids as a group do have more of a tendency to have a learning disability in addition to their ADHD. In the general population, 5 to 10 percent of all children have learning disabilities.[1] In the ADHD population, this figure is more like 45 percent.[2] Children with ADHD, therefore, often have two challenges to deal with.

> **Key Concept**
> As a group, kids with ADHD are more likely than their peers to have a learning disability.

The result of all these problems is that children with ADHD are often significant underachievers at school. From a very early point in time, they find that they do not like school. A typical conversation with a child with ADHD during a diagnostic evaluation may go something like this:

"What do you think of school?"

"I don't like it."

"What don't you like about it?"

"It's boring."

"What's boring about it?"

"The work."

"What's your favorite subject?"

"Recess."

A child's "academic self-concept"—or what he expects of himself in school—may be formed very early, perhaps by the third grade.[3] For children with ADHD, this may mean they decide early in their academic careers that school is not the place for them to be.

School: ADHD-PI

The inattentive version of a child with ADHD (ADHD-PI) will show many of the same difficulties as the ADHD-C type, but these kids will not struggle much with disruptive behavior. They may quietly fade into the background of the classroom, and no one seems to notice them. If you watch closely, however, you will see a little girl in trouble. She is dreamy and detached. She does not finish her work on time or at all. She is not really following what is going on in class, but it's easy to miss her inattentiveness because she is polite, tries to be cooperative, makes little noise, and causes no trouble.

I have found that inattentive children are often seen as simply being slow learners, in spite of the fact that most have average or above-average intelligence. Their forgetfulness and disorganization, however, are seen as signs of limited intellectual ability rather than as signs of ADHD. The presence of a learning disability or anxiety can further this mistaken impression of the problem. Due to their quiet and gentle natures, though, in the early grades, these children often are not recognized as needing diagnosis and treatment.

> **Key Concept**
>
> Children with ADHD-PI are often seen as simply being slow learners, in spite of the fact that most have average or above-average intelligence.

Home: ADHD-C

Let's imagine a child with ADHD-C didn't have a good day at school. It would be nice if he could come home, put his feet up, and relax a little. Unfortunately, this is often a challenge.

Children with ADHD-C may be the source of frequent disruption in the family and may produce what seems like an endless flood of noise. Sibling rivalry is unusually intense, and the child with ADHD is often the instigator of the trouble. He can be extremely jealous of siblings, often perceiving that they are liked more by their parents than he is.

General discipline is often a problem for parents who have children diagnosed with ADHD. None of their strategies seem to work as well as they did with their other children.

At home, children with ADHD may not remember the rules or their chores or do not follow through with them when asked. When asked to do even minor things, they may have a major tantrum. They are often sloppy. Asking the child to do several things in sequence is usually a lost cause. After requesting that a youngster turn off the TV, hang up his coat, and come to dinner, for example, parents may return ten minutes later to find the child standing immobile, coat in hand, staring at the television.

As the years go on, both children with ADHD and their parents can experience a continual drop in self-esteem and an increase in depression. As we have mentioned, I've often seen that the very first person in the family to get clobbered by the existence of a child with ADHD is not the child: it is the mother. Mom often gets the brunt of the difficult child's behavior. And since we still live in a society that tends to blame parents for everything their kids do, the parents—and especially the mother—may be constantly trying to figure out what happened with their child.

A Bad Day for Mom

To underline this important point, let's take a quick look at what you might call a bad day for Mom. It goes something like this:

Imagine a mom who has a very active four-year old. She's worried that someday he'll kill his little sister, he seems driven by a motor, and he's been kicked out of two preschools. Mom has an 11:00 a.m. appointment with her pediatrician to talk about the situation. The doctor has said over the phone that perhaps the boy is "hyperactive."

At eleven o'clock, Mom enters the doctor's office with her son. The boy hardly moves, he's polite, he's cute, and he answers all the doctor's questions. Mom is angry, thinking to herself, *What's your problem, kiddo! Do to him what you do to me all the time!* Unfortunately, this physician doesn't know that research has demonstrated that 80 percent of children with ADHD will sit still in a doctor's office.[4]

The doctor's conclusion? Mom may be emotionally unstable or may in fact be causing the boy's bad behavior. The doctor tries to explain this nicely to the mother. Mom is crushed. Her self-esteem drops to -48. She leaves very upset. Children with ADHD-C are not known for their sympathy. Sensing his mother's turmoil, the little fellow acts up worse than ever during the afternoon. This culminates in a full-blown tantrum over a cookie at 6:00 p.m. right as Dad walks in the kitchen door.

Dad sees what's happening and bellows at his son, "Knock it off, young man, or I'll kick your butt from here to Alaska!" Slowly and quietly, the four-year old gets up and slinks out of the kitchen. Dad now turns to Mom, points a finger in her face, and says, "Now why the hell can't you do that!?" Mom's self-esteem at this point? -88.

Not an unusual scenario. Ask the moms of kids with ADHD.

Home: ADHD-PI

In general, children with inattentive ADHD at home are not aggressive disruptors or noisemakers. They may have a mild-mannered disposition and be fairly easy to get along with. Some of these children are actually too passive. They may appear unmotivated and slow to process information. Often, you find they are not listening to you even when you are speaking right to them. They are amazingly forgetful and absentminded. They have trouble getting organized and following through on activities like getting up and out in the morning, doing homework, or completing their chores.

However, children with ADHD-PI do all this quietly and passively. They will not intrude so much on their parents' senses or consciousness. Parents may have to track their little daydreamer down to find out what he or she has or has not accomplished. These children are also more passive in sibling rivalry, but occasionally, they can put up a first-class fuss when they feel they are being treated unfairly or abused. Parents who tend to be well-organized themselves or those who lean toward being perfectionists can certainly find children with ADHD-PI very frustrating, even when making noise or causing major disturbances are pretty much absent in the child's behavior.

Peers: ADHD-C

As if these problems weren't enough, when rambunctious children with ADHD go out and play, they will encounter further difficulties. Their frequent lapses in self-control make it hard to engage in games that require following rules and self-restraint. The child with ADHD suffers from a major case of "low frustration tolerance." Everything is a big deal to them, and they are extremely competitive, often trying to modify or create rules to serve their goal of winning at all cost.

As mentioned before, children with this type of ADHD may often be bossy and sometimes physically aggressive. Parents may be distressed by their child's treatment of playmates who come over to the house. The hyperactive and impulsive child has a very difficult time sharing and does not pay enough attention to what other children want to do. After a difficult few hours, many of the playmates don't want to return again. Some children with ADHD find that other kids do not reciprocate and invite them over to their house. It is not unusual for children with ADHD to be left out of birthday parties that otherwise involve their entire class from school.

Adding to the child's woes is his tendency to get overstimulated in groups and to act "hyper" and silly, making noises, poking people, and being a nuisance. Since kids with ADHD are notoriously insensitive to verbal and nonverbal social cues, many do not realize how poorly they are coming across. Adults who try to tell children with ADHD to "calm down" in these situations find that their words are like throwing gasoline on a fire. Often, the best strategy is to take these children out of the situation for a while to help them calm down.

Although you wouldn't expect it with all these problems, children with ADHD often initiate interactions with other kids, but often in a negative or irritating way. One third-grade girl who was a patient of mine kicked all the boys in the shins in the coat room at the end of the day. It was kind of her way of saying, "See you later, have a nice evening," but the effects were obviously detrimental to her chances of getting along with anybody.

When inevitable fights and arguments do occur, children with ADHD usually blame the other kids for the problem. Parents often try to point out to their children with ADHD-C what they may have done to cause the trouble. However, these corrective explanations don't seem to sink in and often they just irritate the child further.

The result of all these social difficulties is that either children with ADHD-C wind up isolated, or they frequently wind up playing with younger children. The cause for the isolation is obvious, but why do children with ADHD end up playing with children younger than them? There are several reasons.

First, the maturity level of a child with ADHD is usually several years less than his actual chronological age, so he fits in better in that respect. This is often called the "30 Percent Rule."[5] A twelve-year-old child with ADHD-C, for example, will often show the behavioral and emotional maturity of a typically-developing eight- to nine-year-old (30% x 12 years = 3.6; 12 - 3.6 = 8.4 years)

Second, children with ADHD-C are often physically larger than the younger children they tend to spend time with, so the younger ones will let them be the boss. This suits children with ADHD just fine, since they are much less frustrated when they get their way. Younger children often find older children entertaining and fun. Children with ADHD-C always seem to be coming up with something interesting to do. It may not always be good behavior, but if they get caught, the child with ADHD usually takes the rap. This is not to say that it is bad for children with ADHD to play with younger children. It is certainly preferable to not having anyone to play with.

Some children with ADHD also get along better with older kids or children of the opposite sex. These situations can have positive effects. The acid test of the current social skills of children with ADHD, however, is his or her ability to get along with same-age, same-sex children.

In general, children with ADHD are more likely to be rejected by their peer groups because of annoying, aggressive, emotionally intense, and intrusive behavior. They are less likely to have positive reciprocal friendships, and their negative reputations are resistant to change. Even the friendships these kids do have are more likely to be more negative than positive in character, meaning that they are often not strong or entirely pleasant, and they are less stable over time.

Peers: ADHD-PI

Children who have the predominantly inattentive type of ADHD are often overlooked by other children, but they also leave a negative impression on peers.[6] Instead of being pushy and aggressive, they hold back and remain on the fringe of activities, only joining in when they are invited. When they do join an activity, forgetfulness and daydreaming may put them in embarrassing situations. One little boy was playing left field during a baseball game, but he became distracted by a family of geese walking off to his right. As he meandered in their direction, a triple was hit to his left. It took quite a bit of teammates' screaming to bring him back to the game and to his job of retrieving the ball.

Many children with inattentive ADHD, on the other hand, are just fine playmates. They are easygoing, listen fairly well, accommodate others' interests, and often let others direct their play. As opposed to children with ADHD-C, I believe that kids with ADHD-PI may have an advantage when it comes to social skills training. Which is easier to overcome: a bad reputation or almost no reputation? The answer is the latter. Children with ADHD with few black marks against them socially can often be trained to join activities successfully.

3
GROWING UP WITH ADHD

AS THEY PROGRESS FROM infants to adults, children with ADHD will show different characteristics and behaviors at different stages of their development. Life, after all, makes new and unique demands on kids as they get older. Ages three and four, for example, require mastering self-care skills, such as getting dressed, tying shoes, and brushing teeth. Ages eight and nine ask that children make and keep friends, clean their room, and finish homework. The interaction of ADHD symptoms with life's demands will produce a constantly changing picture as a child grows up. Unfortunately, ADHD often interferes with developmental tasks, and as individuals get older, of course, life almost always demands more and more self-control.

Not all children with ADHD will show every single one of the characteristics or problems I discuss in this chapter. The developmental course I first describe represents what you might expect of a typical child with an ADHD combined presentation (ADHD-C), where no diagnosis or effective treatment has been undertaken. Then we will take a look at the case of Sarah, a girl who grew up with undetected ADHD predominantly inattentive presentation (ADHD-PI).

As you read these two developmental descriptions, keep in mind that an accurate and detailed developmental history is one of the most important parts of a good diagnostic evaluation for ADHD.

Developmental Course: ADHD-C

Infancy

The infant signs listed here correlate to some extent with ADHD-C, but they are not as reliable as those indicators that will be described later. There is a tendency for infants who are later diagnosed with ADHD to show more "regulatory issues" such as persistent crying, sleeping issues, and feeding problems.[1]

Keep in mind that these infant signs should be taken with a grain of salt. Many kids with ADHD were fairly peaceful babies, and not every fussy or restless infant will grow up to have an ADHD diagnosis.

Toddler Years

More reliable indicators of ADHD occur when babies become toddlers. In fact, experts believe that it is possible to identify many children with ADHD by age three or four.[2] The predominant indicators, though, will not include short attention span, because few three-year-olds concentrate on anything for very long.

Instead, noncompliance can become more of a problem, and stubbornness may be extreme. If the child is a firstborn, it is difficult for parents to tell if their child is just going through the "terrible twos." The child may walk early and always be on the go. Many of these children are accident-prone due to their hyperactivity, impulsivity, and the frequent coordination difficulties that many of them experience. They often stop taking naps at an early age—much to the chagrin of their mothers. They demand attention, and they do not play well alone. If there are other children in the household, sibling rivalry and jealousy can be constant and extremely intense.

Ages Three to Five

As children with ADHD get older, noncompliance in public can become more of an issue, very often creating extremely embarrassing situations for the parents. Many families simply stop going out together very much or even taking vacations because of the awful scenes they have been through in cars, restaurants, and motels.

Peer problems can also emerge as children graduate from parallel play to more interactive play, where the situational demands to share, listen, and get along are greater. Phone calls from preschools and kindergartens about the child's misbehavior may begin. It is not unusual to find kids with ADHD who have already been kicked out of one or more preschools, often because of their aggressive behavior and difficulty complying with the normal routines.

At this age, it also becomes more obvious that discipline doesn't work with children with ADHD in the same way it does with other children, and discipline may inspire fits of temper that are totally out of proportion to the actual difficulty. Hostile destructiveness is not uncommon during this age range, but children with ADHD can also break or dismantle things simply out of impulsive childlike curiosity.

Another interesting correlate of ADHD I have found is that household pets, such as dogs and cats, often avoid young children with ADHD who are consistently too rough with them. Animals naturally avoid repeating painful experiences.

During these years, parents may start arguing more and more about how to handle children with ADHD, causing increased, regular marital friction. The fact that children with ADHD, discipline-wise, often respond better to their fathers (as most kids do) than to their mothers usually doesn't help the situation. A number of studies have shown the divorce and separation rates to be higher in families that have children with ADHD.[3]

Ages Five to Twelve

Symptoms of ADHD combined presentation really become a problem when children are between the ages of five and twelve. Demands to sit still and concentrate increase dramatically in first grade, which is especially challenging for children with ADHD-C.

Retention—holding the child back a year in school—may also be considered around this time, because children with ADHD are often perceived as immature. Retention should be given careful thought, however. Holding a child back can be a big mistake unless a complete ADHD evaluation is done. If the problem is primarily ADHD and nothing is done to treat the condition, many of these kids will create just as much trouble the second time around in first grade.

In the first, second, and third grades, problems with learning disabilities may begin to emerge, since a large portion (about 45 percent) of children with ADHD will also have a learning disability.[4] In addition, it is very common for kids with ADHD to have problems with handwriting. For many of them, this is because they rush their work (hyperactivity plus impulsivity), but it is also often because their fine motor coordination isn't as developed as that of their peers. Certain subjects, like math and reading, demand a high level of sustained concentration, and these are often areas where ADHD causes great difficulty.

Socially, the child with ADHD may not have a lot—if any—friends, and misbehavior such as lying, fighting, and stealing can increase. Lying is often related to unfinished schoolwork. Trends toward acting out are worrisome, because we know that about 50–60 percent of children with ADHD will also quality for oppositional defiant disorder (ODD).[5] These kids with ADHD and ODD are at serious risk for later developing conduct disorder (CD), the modern euphemism for juvenile delinquency—problems that involve more serious, age-inappropriate, and precocious activities that are sometimes illegal.[6]

During the elementary school years, children with ADHD are old enough to know something is wrong in their life, and their parents may begin to worry about their child developing low self-esteem. Does low self-esteem in fact develop in the child? Those of us who have worked with children with ADHD over the years have noticed, rather than appearing to suffer from low self-esteem, these children appear to think unrealistically highly of themselves.

Though they are not delusional, children with ADHD-C (and perhaps ADHD-PI) often describe friends they don't really have and academic success they have not achieved. When trouble does occur, what comes out of their mouths is often an attempt to blame parents, teachers, or other kids for the problems. This tendency toward overly positive self-perceptions is called *positive illusory bias*, and some see it as a kind of self-protective mechanism for these children.

Adolescence

ADHD and adolescence often don't mix well. While I have found that many children with ADHD will simmer down some in terms of gross motor restlessness (hyperactivity), much of the time, ADHD-C in the thirteen- to nineteen-year-old crowd means adolescence with a vengeance.

By the time children with ADHD becomes teenagers, many families are fed up with their child's behavior and at the end of their rope after years of frustration. Other family members, especially fathers, can themselves sometimes get mad—seemingly at the drop of a hat—and occasionally outdo their own child's tantrums. Parents get especially frustrated with their child's arguing. For years, children with ADHD had to have the last word, never took no for an answer, and argued endlessly over the slightest issues.

As for school, many teenagers with ADHD are sick of school by the time they hit ninth grade. Academically, they may be significantly behind their peers due to all the years when they couldn't concentrate enough to learn what they were supposed to be learning. Tackling high school courses with this shaky base—on top of the residual attention problem—is, of course, extremely difficult. Though most of these kids with ADHD will graduate from high school, they are more likely to fail courses and have lower levels of class placement than their peers.[7]

Difficulties with their peers can continue in adolescence, although these problems may not be as severe as they were when the child was younger, more aggressive, and bossier. Isolation, however, is frequently a problem, or the teen may go through a series of short-term relationships with friends or romantic partners that just never seem to last. A frequent concern of parents is that their teenager does have friends but the parents either don't like them or rarely get a chance to meet them. Parents worry that their unsuccessful teenager with ADHD will hang out with the "stoner" crowd—those kids who also don't like teachers, school, and parents.

There is also now plenty of research evidence that teens with ADHD are not as good at driving as other teenagers who do not have ADHD.[8] (Non-ADHD teens, of course, especially males, are not such good drivers in the first place!) Teens with ADHD get more speeding tickets, have more accidents, have worse accidents than their peers, and are more likely to have their licenses revoked.[9]

Imagine an adolescent with ADHD driving to the store to get in line for a newly released video game. He approaches a light that just turned yellow. Impulsivity, difficulty delaying gratification, emotional overarousal, and noncompliance might all conspire here to produce a dangerous situation—running the yellow. Driving performance is usually not such a horrible problem that one should keep these kids off the road, but many parents set very strict rules about driving, and many push back by a year or two the age at which they allow their kids with ADHD to drive.

Yet the picture is not all bleak for teens with ADHD. Some of them will experience a noticeable drop in hyperactivity and emotional overarousal as they get older, going on to college and finding successful jobs while balancing an exuberant social life. Parents find, though, that teenagers with ADHD always seem to keep them somewhat off-balance.

Adulthood

Approximately two-thirds of children with ADHD grow up to be adults with ADHD.[10] Though this fact is discouraging, the situation is not necessarily bad. True, symptoms like concentration difficulties, emotional overarousal, and even some forms of impulsivity can continue into adulthood. On the other hand, even though some symptoms continue, they do tend to become less severe than in the person's younger years. Gross motor hyperactivity will diminish quite a bit, perhaps partly because the adult has many more pounds to maneuver around.

Though the symptoms that characterize childhood ADHD-C may

lessen, secondary problems that were not part of the original picture may now have come along for the ride. These problems can include anxiety, depression, and substance abuse. As one might expect from the basic symptom profile, adults with ADHD also have more difficulties in the workplace. These include

> **Key Concept**
> Approximately two-thirds of children with ADHD grow up to be adults with ADHD.

reduced productivity, more accidents, and higher absenteeism.[11]

One significant blessing for many adults with ADHD is that there is no more school! Unless, of course, by choice, but now there's a difference: adults with ADHD choose to attend school and are no longer going for the benefit of their parents or society. They can choose a subject they are more interested in, and—as we have seen— interest value can help both attention and motivation considerably.

Adults with ADHD may choose not to go to school anymore. Enough is enough! They may instead pick an occupation that better suits their skills and temperament. The personalities of some adults with ADHD may actually make them more effective in their work. Although difficulty paying attention is rarely an asset, some of the other ADHD symptoms may be an asset in some kinds of work.

Someone who is reasonably intelligent and has good social skills, an intense energy level, strong emotions, and aggressiveness (when appropriate) can certainly succeed in certain jobs. Some may be good entrepreneurs and may succeed at starting their own businesses. They will do better in situations where they don't have a boss. Others may do well at outside sales, where they can drive around or travel, meet different people, and use their energy to close deals. The bad news for salespeople with ADHD? From time to time, they are required to sit down at a desk and write their weekly or monthly activity or expense report!

Many adults who maintain some of their ADHD symptoms will be employed, in relationships, physically healthy, and self-supporting. The symptoms they do maintain are usually treatable.

Developmental Course: ADHD-PI

Now that we've described a typical developmental path for the ADHD combined category, let's take a look the life of Sarah. Sarah will give us some insight into ADHD predominantly inattentive.

Sarah's mother said Sarah was an easy baby. She seemed to have a very pleasant, calm temperament, smiling often and enjoying the presence of other people. Her developmental milestones were normal. Sarah walked at about twelve months and was putting a few words together just after age two.

During her preschool years, Sarah presented no particular problems. Her mother went back to work when Sarah was about three. For about three to four weeks, however, Sarah had trouble separating from her mom when she was dropped off at day care. She did not have tantrums, but she cried and was reluctant to go inside. Of course, this reaction made her mother feel guilty about going to work. She often thought about her daughter during the day and sometimes called the center. At those times, she was told Sarah was doing fine.

Socially, Sarah seemed to enjoy the presence of other children, but she also seemed somewhat passive and hesitant. When first introduced to a new group of kids, she just watched and listened, standing off to the side. She obviously enjoyed the other children, though, because she smiled and laughed at the children as they played. Gradually, Sarah got more involved, especially if she was not forced to do so before she was ready. Fortunately, her parents and teachers appreciated the fact that it was not a good idea to push her in this way.

Sarah loved kindergarten, and she especially loved her teacher, Mrs. MacArthur. The feeling was reciprocal, because Sarah was also one of Mrs. MacArthur's favorites. She kept telling Sarah's parents that their little girl was "so sweet!" Sarah was a sweet kid. She often seemed to be in good spirits, rarely got mad, and never caused any trouble. She was always willing to help and cooperate with any agenda. Sarah also seemed to be progressing socially and had two good friends she played with every day.

Sarah: Elementary School

In first grade, things went okay for a while, but not quite as well as kindergarten. According to her teacher, Sarah sometimes appeared "a little slower than the other children." She had trouble keeping her pencils and papers in order, and she also frequently lost things. Her teacher also commented that Sarah "was not always with the rest of the class." Sometimes, she was looking out the window, and at other times, she seemed lost in a daydream.

In November, Sarah resisted going to school again. She had trouble leaving the house on time to catch the bus. When her dad asked her if she liked school, she said yes but without as much enthusiasm as she had shown in kindergarten. This stage quickly passed, and Sarah's parents were reassured that there was a lot of variation among first graders.

Concerns began to arise in second and third grades, however. Teachers commented more often about Sarah's disorganization and inability to focus on the task at hand. Yet as soon as any teacher uttered these criticisms, the words were followed with the comment, "But don't worry, everything will be fine. She's such a sweet girl."

Sarah was still a sweet girl. At home, she gave her parents little trouble, except she couldn't seem to remember to do her chores, she had a hard time getting up and out the door in the morning, and she was always losing things. Sarah's parents didn't get overly concerned about this, and their daughter's pleasant disposition made it hard to get mad at her.

As elementary school progressed, Sarah stumbled along. Once letter grades appeared on the report card, she got mostly Cs, with an occasional D or B. Teachers' comments about Sarah's inattentiveness, disorganization, and problems completing work continued. All her teachers liked her though. They all felt she wanted to cooperate, and her failings were simply due to some kind of absentmindedness. Sarah didn't present any behavior problems, and she seemed to get along well with the other children.

Sarah in Middle and High School

Sarah struggled considerably more in middle school where she had seven different teachers and a lot more homework. Her organizational skills, which had never been strong, were at this point overwhelmed. She brought the wrong books to the wrong classes. She lost her assignments. Term papers and other long-term projects were forgotten until the last minute. Her parents were now beginning to wonder if their daughter wasn't being just a little bit obstinate. Arguments about school and schoolwork increased. Homework took Sarah three to four hours a night to complete, and even then, the work was hurried, messy, and full of careless mistakes.

In eighth grade, something happened that changed Sarah's life. Her English teacher asked her to read a poem in front of the whole class. She wasn't crazy about the idea, but she walked up to the front of the room. While she was reading, however, she began feeling short of breath, and she started sweating. Her hands began to shake, and she could hardly hold the paper. Her voice shook. She wanted to run away, but she couldn't. She felt like a total fool.

Finally, the teacher quietly asked Sarah if she was okay. Sarah said she didn't know, and her teacher told her she didn't have to finish. Sarah sat down, completely humiliated. She couldn't look at anybody. After class, her teacher tried to talk to her, but Sarah hurried away.

Sarah had been blindsided by her first panic attack, induced by a fairly common fear—the fear of public speaking. She hoped at first that it had just been a bad day. But the next time she had to read or speak in class, she panicked again. From then on, she dreaded going to school, horrified by the thought that she might be called on to once again make a fool out of herself in front of everybody.

Sarah's anxiety added to her inattentiveness. Her grades dropped further in high school. Now she was getting Cs, Ds, and Fs. Her parents grew more frustrated with her. They were always asking her what was the matter, but Sarah simply said she didn't know. Her anxiety generalized into social situations. She was now afraid to speak up in any group and never wanted to be the center of attention. Speech class was total terror. She feared people would hear her voice quaver or see her hands shake. She couldn't drink coffee in front of anyone or even hold a soup spoon. She only brought things for lunch like sandwiches, which she could grab with both hands, or else, she just didn't eat.

As Sarah's anxiety increased and her school performance got worse, her self-esteem plummeted. She became more and more depressed. She had little contact with friends. Finally, her parents took her to see a psychologist. Sarah thought this was even more embarrassing than her first speech. Although Dr. Walker was a very nice woman, Sarah said very little, and she did not mention her problem with anxiety. The psychologist concluded the girl was depressed, and she recommended counseling and medication.

Sarah started seeing Dr. Walker weekly. She also began taking a medication that Dr. Walker described as an antidepressant. After a month or so, to her surprise, Sarah did start feeling better. She also began feeling less anxious, which relieved her. One day, she actually gave a speech at school without any symptoms of panic.

Finally, Sarah told Dr. Walker about her problem with panicky feelings during social situations and public speaking. Dr. Walker explained that the medication was probably helping with her anxiety too, which was exactly what was happening.

But Sarah's schoolwork continued to be a problem. Her grades had improved to Cs with an occasional D. She still hated homework, and long-term assignments were torture as usual. Dr. Walker and her parents felt she was brighter than these grades indicated, so psychological testing was ordered. Sarah came up with a full-scale IQ of 123. She was bright!

So why the average to below-average grades? No one could figure it out. The focus on depression, and later on anxiety, had helped to cover the existence of ADHD-PI.

Sarah muddled through two years at a community college; her grades didn't improve. By that time, she was sick of school and wanted to do just about anything else. She started working at a fast-food restaurant. Although the work was boring and the manager sometimes got after her for forgetting some of her jobs, it was still better than school.

Eventually Sarah married Mark, one of the managers at the restaurant. Although he was almost ten years older than she, they had one thing in common: they were both shy. Sarah had stopped taking the antidepressant, and a good deal of her social anxiety had returned, but Mark let her avoid working the cash register because of her trembling hands. Mark understood her reluctance.

At first, being married didn't seem so bad. Mark and Sarah agreed that she could stay home for a while and not have to work. Sarah had two babies in just under three years.

Conclusions

Among the many conclusions that can be drawn from the above developmental histories, several stand out.

First, children with ADHD-PI are usually hard or impossible to distinguish from non-ADHD preschool kids. All preschoolers show fairly short attention spans.

Second, disruptive behavior (restlessness, running excessively, noisiness, blurting out, and interrupting) drives referrals for evaluation, especially in schools. In other words, the kids with ADHD who are most likely to be diagnosed early are the children with ADHD-C—the ones that are always "in your face." Inattentive youngsters, like Sarah, are often diagnosed later, or worse, never evaluated at all.

> **Key Concept**
>
> The older a child with ADHD gets, the more likely it becomes that he or she will also develop another psychological disorder.

Third, the older a child with ADHD gets, the more likely it becomes that he or she will also develop another psychological disorder. As adults, over 80 percent of individuals with ADHD have one additional disorder, over 50 percent have two additional disorders, and over 33 percent have three.[12] Sarah eventually had trouble with anxiety and then depression. Anxiety and depression are what are often called internalizing disorders—they do not directly bother anyone other than the person afflicted with them. As an individual gets older, anxiety and depression will often accompany both ADHD-PI as well as ADHD-C.[13]

4
CAUSES OF ADHD

WHAT CAUSES ADHD? PERHAPS we should first clarify the question. What we are really asking is this: what causes a chronic behavioral pattern characterized by inattentiveness, impulsivity, and hyperactivity? Or, if we look at ADHD as a problem with self-control, we are asking: what could cause persistent problems with response inhibition and other executive functions such as working memory, internal language, and emotional regulation?

Questions about causes of ADHD can also be answered at different levels. Is ADHD hereditary? If so, what type of vulnerability is passed on from parent to child? Is it a chemical imbalance of some kind, or a structural difference in the brain? If ADHD is not hereditary, what factors might produce it? Is it a learned effect of bad parenting? What about stress, brain injury, or impaired fetal development? Let's sort this out.

Hereditary vs. Learned

We have known for some time that ADHD is a disorder that has a powerful hereditary component. ADHD, in other words, is not something you learn as you grow up—even by means of lousy parenting. Look, for example, at these facts:

1. If a parent has ADHD, each of their kids has a 50–50 chance of also having ADHD.[1]
2. Kids' ADHD shows a strong tendency to match both the nature and the severity of their parents' ADHD.[2]
3. If a child has a sibling with ADHD, that child's chances of also having ADHD go from 5–7 percent to about 30 percent.[3]
4. Twin studies reveal that genetics account for about 70–80 percent of the variation in ADHD symptoms. If two twins are raised by different parents, for example, and one twin turns out to have ADHD, there is a better than 50 percent chance that the other twin will also have ADHD.[4]
5. Biological parents of children with ADHD show a much greater prevalence of ADHD themselves than do the adoptive parents of children with ADHD. (It's nice to know that parents can't catch ADHD from their kids!)[5]
6. ADHD is clearly one of the most strongly inherited of all psychiatric disorders, rivaled only by bipolar and autism spectrum disorders.[6]

> **Key Concept**
>
> Twin studies reveal that genetics account for about 70 to 80 percent of the variation in ADHD symptoms.

One of the most important lessons from all this research is this: "bad parenting," such as being overly permissive or overly harsh, does not cause ADHD. If you are a lousy parent, for example, you might contribute to your child's anxiety, depression, or low self-esteem, but you won't make them have ADHD. ADHD is pretty much going to happen if the right genes are there—no matter what you do—and it's not going to happen if that genetic base is not there.

The fact that ADHD is not caused by bad parenting has big implications for treatment, since getting rid of parental guilt helps moms and dads cope a lot better with the problem. But before you get too excited, there are two other things you should know: you can make ADHD worse by bad parenting, and bad parenting can greatly increase the chances of a child with ADHD acquiring two other disorders, oppositional defiance and conduct disorder. This is discussed in greater depth in chapter 8 about treatment.

The Mechanics of Genetics

How do children inherit certain traits from their parents? From high school biology classes, you may remember the studies of Mendel with his peas and his demonstration of how organisms pass down genetic traits to their offspring. Children receive thousands and thousands of genes from their parents. These genes carry instructions for how to make a human being, and they also carry instructions that determine the many specific hereditary traits (height, IQ, skin color) that human beings have.

Genes don't always do their work the way humans might like, and when errors occur, serious problems can sometimes result. Errors in single genes, for example, are known to cause thousands of hereditary diseases. These include cystic fibrosis and Huntington's chorea, a severe, degenerative neurological disorder. Other disorders can occur when there are problems with several genes at the same time. These are called complex genetic disorders, and they often interact with environmental factors to produce certain results. Most psychiatric problems, cancer, and heart disease fall into the category of complex genetic disorders.

It is likely that ADHD falls into this last category as well. Most experts feel that several of the one hundred thousand or so human genes will eventually be implicated in the occurrence of ADHD, rather than just one.[7] Researchers are hot on the trail of genetic variations or abnormalities that tend to run in families where ADHD is present.[8] One recent list of suspected genes included forty-four different possibilities, with names like TPH1, ADRAIA, NFIL3, SLC6A3, and DRD1.[9]

Genetic research, however, often gets ahead of actual treatment. Simply knowing which genes do what does not automatically lead to an effective way of dealing with a problem. Researchers are also focusing on how these genes interact with the environment—in other words, how the genes are expressed. Genetic research is an exciting development in the field of ADHD.

ADHD and the Brain

To say that a disorder is hereditary does not really explain what is causing the problem on any given day. It simply means that whatever is causing the problem can be passed on from generation to generation. There's another important question: what is going on in this person right now that produces ADHD symptoms?

Today, more and more people are referring to ADHD as a neurobiological condition. That's because more and more research is pointing out that problems with attention, impulse control, activity level, and self-regulation result from the inadequate functioning of certain areas of the brain.

One of the areas of the brain that appears to be frequently involved in ADHD is known as the prefrontal cortex. The prefrontal cortex, with its connections to other brain areas, is associated with both behavioral inhibition (the ability to stop, look, and listen) and the other executive functions mentioned earlier.

Several lines of research have implicated the prefrontal cortex:

▸ Glucose metabolism studies (PET scans) have shown that these prefrontal areas of the brain are actually underactive in subjects with ADHD.
▸ The prefrontal areas of the brain are dopamine-rich areas, and we know that our most potent anti-ADHD medications (the stimulants) enhance dopamine functioning.
▸ Recent neuroimaging studies have suggested that these brain regions are smaller than normal in persons with ADHD.[10]

So it looks like what's passed on genetically with ADHD is a predisposition for the prefrontal cortex to not be able to do its job well. People often wonder "Why in the world would you give a stimulant medication to a hyperactive person?" Now you can begin to understand the reason: with ADHD, parts of the brain (prefrontal cortex) that play a significant role in regulating a person's activities are actually underactive. These parts of the central nervous system, in other words, must be stimulated in order to do their job right.

Imagine, for example, that the governor of a state was lazy, drank constantly, and spent all day in bed. The state itself would be a mess. People would fight, rob each other, not pay taxes. The schools, police, post office, and other services would be terribly inefficient. Social, economic, and political chaos would result, and everyone would be miserable.

But imagine you could get that governor out of bed, take him over to the window, and say, "Look what's going on out there!" Perhaps you could stimulate him to do his job better, with the result that the state would become more orderly. Crime would drop, people would pay their taxes, the mail would get delivered, and generally, people would be a lot happier.

The evidence suggests that something analogous to that occurs in the central nervous system of persons with ADHD.[11] Deficiencies in the prefrontal cortex (and its connections with other brain centers) result in a kind of lazy governor, with the result that the activities of the individual with ADHD are random, unfocused, disorganized, sometimes too aggressive, and frequently overly emotional. The person does whatever he or she feels like doing at the moment. Self-restraint and future goals are sacrificed.

Stimulant medications, however, can stimulate the lazy prefrontal cortex in the brain to do its job right, with the result that the activities of the person with ADHD become more focused, organized, and purposeful.

So current research indicates that ADHD has something to do with a predominantly inherited *inability* of the prefrontal areas of the brain to do their job of self-regulation correctly. Yet heredity may not be the whole story for everyone who has ADHD.

Studies have also shown that ADHD can be related to biological hazards that can affect brain development before, during, or after birth.[12] Identifiable risk factors include maternal smoking, maternal alcohol use, prematurity, lead levels in the body, and low birth weight. These hazards may somehow impact the prefrontal areas of the developing brain in the fetus. Brain injury to children and adults has also produced symptoms that are very similar to ADHD.

It is now estimated that acquired cases of ADHD, in which adverse environmental influences affect brain development, may account for up to 35 percent of the total prevalence of this disorder.[13] Though these dangers contribute to ADHD less than heredity, unlike genetic causes, they are largely preventable.

ADHD and Bad Parenting

There are plenty of bad parents in the world. Some are grossly negligent, some are sexually or physically abusive, and some are just plain mean. It is highly unlikely, though, that any of them ever singlehandedly caused ADHD in one or more of their children. Children do not learn to have ADHD. You can certainly cause psychological problems in your kids by bad parenting, but ADHD isn't one of them.

Unfortunately, I believe that the notion that "screwy parents make screwy kids" is still a widely held view of child-rearing in our society. This idea might be called the psychological, psychogenic, or family dynamic theory of ADHD, and it produces a great deal of unnecessary guilt in parents of kids with ADHD. In our schools, I have found the psychogenic view is still the predominant theory regarding childhood emotional and behavioral problems. Parents of kids with ADHD find this idea subtly—and sometimes overtly—expressed in the comments and reactions of friends, pediatricians, psychologists, teachers, and relatives. The message is something like this: "If you would only set firmer limits [or "argued less," or "drank less," or "spent more time at home," and so on], that little brat of yours would act like a normal child." Many parents, of course, blame themselves for their challenging child's behavior long before anyone else does. It's important to remember: ADHD is primarily hereditary, and the other factors that may also cause ADHD (or something like it) are biological hazards. ADHD is not caused by bad parenting.

Bad parenting, however, can affect a child with ADHD in two important ways. First, because of the genetic aspect of ADHD, many parents of diagnosed children have ADHD (as well as other disorders) themselves, and it is often hard for them to be reasonable and consistent.[14] That is why in order for the treatment of a child with ADHD to be effective, it often must involve the concurrent treatment of one or both parents.

Second, bad parenting can contribute to comorbidity—the development of additional psychiatric problems. We can look at comorbidity in two ways by examining what are called externalizing and internalizing disorders. Externalizing disorders, such as ADHD, oppositional defiant disorder (ODD), and conduct disorder (CD) don't bother the person who has them as much as they bother other people and society. Externalizing disorders can also be thought of as "garlic" problems. Internalizing disorders (anxiety, depression) bother the person who has them, but not necessarily other people.

On the externalizing side, we know that marital instability and poor parenting can facilitate the metamorphosis of ADHD and ODD into CD. CD, in turn can result in an adult version of the problem known as antisocial personality disorder (ASPD). People with ASPD lack empathy, are callous and cynical, take advantage of others, and feel little guilt.

On the internalizing side, anxiety and depression will at least be exacerbated—if not caused—by a parent who is constantly nagging, lecturing, or screaming at a child. Anxiety and depression can also be worsened by constant marital bickering and fighting.

The moral of the story is this: your parenting weaknesses didn't cause your child to have ADHD. On the other hand, if you have a child with ADHD, you'd better work hard on these weaknesses for your sake and the sake of your kids.

What *Doesn't* Cause ADHD?

Diet does not produce ADHD. Systematic research has consistently failed to support the idea that artificial colorings, flavorings, or natural salicylates are troublemakers that produce ADHD or learning disabilities (LD) in children.[15] However, it may be true that there is a very small group of kids who are diet-sensitive in some ways, as evidenced by the existence of an entire chapter in Russell A. Barkley's *Attention-Deficit Hyperactivity Disorder*. So parents' claims to that effect should never be taken lightly.

Also, contrary to popular belief, *sugar* doesn't cause hyperactivity either. Some interesting studies have shown that children who eat too much sugar actually reduce their hyperactivity, but it also hurts their concentration.[16]

However, many parents steadfastly claim that their child with ADHD goes crazy after consuming too much sugar. If your child has this reaction, limiting sugar intake certainly makes sense. Make sure, though, that it's the sugar that made her hyper, and not the situation—such as a wild and crazy birthday party!

In a way similar to the dietary effects we just discussed, *allergies* may aggravate ADHD, but they don't produce this disorder to start with.[17] A child who is allergic and feeling sick is very likely to be more irritable, oppositional, and generally out of sorts. Unfortunately, studies have shown that children with ADHD are more prone to allergies than the rest of the population.[18] So it's quite possible for a child to have ADHD and be allergic. The symptoms of allergies can complicate ADHD behavior, and so can some of the medications used to treat them.

> **Key Concept**
>
> Contrary to popular belief, sugar doesn't cause hyperactivity.

People often ask: "Why is there so much ADHD around now compared to previous years? Is there some new factor that is causing a dramatic increase in its prevalence?" The best answer is that ADHD has probably always been around and probably to the same degree it is now. The reason it's being diagnosed more is due to a tremendous increase in public awareness of the problem.

5
PREDICTING THE FUTURE

KIDS WITH ADHD CAN put a lot of stress on their parents. When Johnny flunks his spelling test, refuses to do his homework, lies to cover a mistake, or pushes his sister to the floor, parents can certainly get stressed out.

Parental strain, however, is not just based on what is actually going on right at the moment. Parents' anguish is often created more by worries about how their child will turn out than by what's happening right now. When a child acts up, parents frequently entertain worrisome fantasies about their child never being able to hold a job, needing to live at home well into adulthood, or winding up in prison. These worries may vary from parent to parent, but they often take an extreme form: *imagining the worst*. Such thoughts, consequently, make parents very upset.

Raising a child with ADHD is difficult enough without adding unnecessary worry. Although ADHD is a serious challenge, the future is usually not as bleak as some parents imagine. Most children with ADHD will grow up to be self-supporting adults. Research on ADHD has come up with a number of factors that have been shown to be related to how children with ADHD will turn out as adults. Some of these factors parents can control; others are not under parental control.

Socioeconomic Status (SES)

Higher is better. For a long time, we have known that higher SES is correlated with better physical and mental health.[1] There may be several reasons why a higher family SES leads to a better outcome in a child with ADHD. Perhaps parents in higher socioeconomic brackets are better educated and therefore more aware of potential problems. Perhaps they are more willing to seek assistance in evaluating difficulties with their children. In addition, these parents may be more able to afford diagnosis and treatment and to sustain these efforts over the many years necessary with a child with ADHD.

As mentioned earlier, there is also some association between ADHD and prenatal, perinatal, or postnatal difficulties. The child whose parents are in a higher economic bracket is less likely to experience danger here, because his or her medical care is likely to be of higher quality.

On the other hand, children forced to grow up under conditions of urban poverty experience many risks that can aggravate ADHD and worsen prognosis. Population density, inadequate housing, limited access to health care and other resources, high rates of crime, exposure to biological hazards, and family instability can all increase the risk for psychiatric disorders.

Intelligence (IQ)

Higher is better. In my experience, a bright child with ADHD has a distinct advantage over his less intelligent counterparts. Superior intelligence can go a long way toward compensating for many different challenges, including attention problems and learning disabilities. Since one of the most challenging environments for children with ADHD is school, and since performance in school is very much related to brain power, it is easy to see how a higher IQ can contribute to a better prognosis.

Imagine two different children diagnosed with ADHD. One has an IQ of 100, which is average, or the equivalent of the fiftieth percentile for his age group. The second child has an IQ of 130, which is classified as superior and means this child is smarter than about 97 percent of his own age group. (Keep in mind that an IQ is not a perfect pinpoint-type of score but only an estimate of the child's overall ability.)

Furthermore, let's suppose that these two children are in the same third-grade class, and they are both given the same math problem to do. Having ADHD, they both have a fairly low frustration tolerance, so let's also assume both of them can work on a problem for a maximum of seven minutes before getting frustrated and quitting. The child with the IQ of 130 finishes the math problem in four minutes, feels good about his accomplishment, and receives praise from his teacher. The child with the IQ of 100 is capable of doing this particular problem in ten minutes, but that exceeds his frustration tolerance. After seven minutes of working, he gives up, starts bothering the child next to him, and gets in trouble with the teacher.

Quite different outcomes! Although the example is oversimplified, it gives a fairly clear idea of the advantage IQ can provide a child with ADHD. Multiply these experiences hundreds of times every year for each child, and you can easily imagine the long-term effects.

One caution with bright children with ADHD: these kids are often underdiagnosed. There is a myth that children with ADHD don't get good grades. Bright children with ADHD sometimes coast through the K–5 years with excellent grades. After all, brighter students will find school more interesting, they will be more successful, and they will get positive feedback. Even troublesome ADHD behavior can be somewhat subdued when a child is interested in what he or she is doing. But come middle school and high school, many of these smart children start to slip. Why? Students get more homework, and they have more independence, but they also need more self-control and better organizational skills.

Aggressiveness

Higher is worse. A large percentage of children with ADHD are overly aggressive in social situations. Physical aggression—especially in younger children—may occur, as well as just plain bossiness. Aggressive behavior is fairly common in two- to three-year-olds, so it doesn't always mean there is an unusual problem. Aggression (hitting, kicking, biting, spitting) is much more of a concern when it continues to age five and beyond.

Aggressive behavior does two things: it gets a youngster into trouble with adults, and it turns off a child's peers. Aggressive behavior—much more than simple inattentiveness—generates referrals for evaluation. In a sense, this is good, because possible ADHD may be discovered. But this kind of behavior is still a big worry. Satterfield, for example, found that both hyperactivity and aggression contributed to the development of criminal behavior in childhood and adolescence.[2] Oppositional defiant behavior, for example, which is usually more reactive than aggressive, when combined with ADHD may evolve into conduct disorder, which is defiant, aggressive, and mean. ADHD/CD kids are a big challenge—and their behavior is hard to change.

Aggressive behavior also makes an unfavorable impression on one's peers, resulting in a bad reputation that is hard to modify. Studies have shown that bad reputations persist in people's minds even though the initial behavior that produced the reputation has changed for the better.[3]

Hyperactivity

Higher is worse. Just as with the level of aggressiveness, the child who is extremely active will run into more problems than his less active counterparts. Although most hyperactive children can sometimes sit still in situations that are novel, interesting, intimidating, or one-on-one with an adult, there are a few children with ADHD who can literally never sit still. Some, for example, cannot sit through a children's TV program where only a short attention span is required. Others cannot stay focused during preschool or kindergarten activities, which are usually short as well as fun. As was mentioned earlier, most children will outgrow their hyperactivity once they reach adolescence, but those few kids who do not are in for more problems.[4]

Ironically, there may be an instance where being less hyperactive is a drawback. This has to do with children with ADHD-PI and perhaps with sluggish cognitive tempo (SCT). Since these children are not as active as those with ADHD-C, and since they are more the "pleasant space cadet" type, they do not come to the attention of the adults who might be able to evaluate and help them. Therefore, as they grow up, they run into more and more problems, their self-esteem drops, and they are more vulnerable to anxiety and depression. But nobody does anything about it, because these children are internalizers—they are causing little trouble for anyone else.

Social Skills

Higher is better. It is a well-established fact that social skills are extremely critical factors in determining a child's future happiness.[5] In his classic work, *Emotional Intelligence*, author Daniel Goleman describes emotional aptitude as a kind of "meta-ability" that explains why one person thrives in life while another does not.[6]

One study, for example, looked at people diagnosed with schizophrenia and at a simple trait known as likability. This investigation concluded that *likeable* schizophrenics had a much better prognosis than *obnoxious* schizophrenics.[7] This research is interesting and somewhat disheartening with respect to ADHD, because kids with ADHD-C engage in a lot of abrasive behavior. It is hard to feel compassion for—or to want to help—someone who is always unpleasant to be with.

Psychologists become very concerned about children with ADHD if they have not developed some reasonable social abilities and do not have some friends by the age of ten. If she is still isolated (as with ADHD-PI) or arguing and fighting a lot with peers (as with ADHD-C), she is in trouble.

Oddly enough, some ADHD characteristics can, periodically, be assets for some children. The hyperactive older child (or adult) can sometimes be the life of the party. He may be enjoyed for his overarousal and high energy level, provided these qualities do not reach ridiculous or irritating proportions. Also, there is sometimes a fine line between bossiness and leadership. Some children with ADHD tend toward bossiness, but they are capable of getting their way in a not-so-abrasive manner, and other kids follow them. This can be an asset. Maybe they'll run their own company someday!

Early Diagnosis

Earlier is better. Detecting just about any problem at the earliest possible stage, whether it's astigmatism, cancer, a learning disability, or ADHD, is always preferable. Young children are still very malleable. If their ADHD is picked up in the preschool years and dealt with properly, these kids have a good chance of developing fairly normally and avoiding major problems. Remember that we think we can detect roughly 70 percent of children with ADHD by about age three (usually ADHD-C).[8] Trying to treat a seventeen-year-old with ADHD for the first time is often very difficult, because the child is so much more likely to be resistant and to have adapted to the way he or she is.

There is another reason early detection is better. If we can pick up ADHD early and treat it appropriately, we may be able to prevent—or eliminate—certain comorbid problems. Pera suggests that the basic elements of successful couples' counseling can be usefully applied to adults with ADHD.[9] When parents have access to these strategies, it can prevent some children with ADHD-C from making the ADHD-to-ODD-to-CD progression. In other children with ADHD-PI, treating ADHD early and thus preventing school failure will very likely prevent later anxiety, depression, and poor self-esteem.

Family Strength

Higher is better. A strong family unit can do a lot to help children with ADHD develop more normally. If a child feels parents and siblings are on his side and care about him, his self-regard will suffer much less from the inevitable battering he will receive in other areas of his life.

If parents can negotiate their differences in a democratic and satisfactory way, especially in regard to the child with ADHD, if the family allows for open expression of thoughts and feelings, and if discipline is handled in a loving but firm manner, the child will be better off.

Physically and psychologically healthy parents make for a more stable and strong family. The more resilient parents are—emotionally and behaviorally—and the better care they take of themselves, the better off the children will be. Unfortunately, it is often hard for parents to show these positive qualities for two reasons: the stress children with ADHD create and the fact that biological parents of children with ADHD have a tendency toward having certain types of psychological problems themselves. That's why treating a child with ADHD usually involves treating the parents as well.

> **Key Concept**
> A strong family unit can do a lot to help children with ADHD develop more typically.

Want a quick and dirty way to diagnose a family's strength? How much fun do these people have with each other? It is unfortunately true that when there is a child with ADHD in a family, family fun can be difficult to orchestrate. Sibling rivalry, for one thing, can ruin many an outing. Although it can be challenging with a child who has ADHD, the family that regularly plays together is always better off. Keep in mind that some of the best times are one-on-one times— one parent and one child enjoying each other's company. One sure strength of individuals with ADHD is their ability to have fun!

Comorbidity

More is usually worse. By the time they are in their teens, less than 50 percent of children with ADHD will be what is sometimes referred to as "squeaky clean" ADHD—that is, the only psychological problem they have is ADHD.[10] The rest of the kids, however, will have at least one other psychological condition in addition to their ADHD. The more challenges a child with ADHD faces, the poorer the prognosis is going to be. These additional problems, which can vary in their own degree of severity, can include conduct disorder (in children and teens), antisocial personality and substance abuse (in teens and adults), anxiety, depression, learning disabilities, and bipolar disorder.

On the other hand, there may occasionally be certain kinds of comorbid anxiety that may actually counteract ADHD to some extent and improve prognosis. For example, ADHD involves impulsive behavior and difficulty with self-restraint. An overly anxious person is the opposite. She is always thinking *What if this happens?* or *What if that happens?* Anxious people are often cautious, reserved, and even inhibited. It's not hard to imagine the anxious tendency counteracting the impulsive tendency, thus reducing chaotic behavior, poorly thought-out decisions, and obnoxious statements.

Overall Severity of ADHD

Higher is worse. ADHD comes in different shades of gray that range from mild to severe in the *DSM-5*. Mild ADHD involves just enough symptoms to make the diagnosis, and these symptoms cause only minor impairments in social, academic, or occupational functioning. Severe ADHD, on the other hand, involves many symptoms in excess of those required to make the diagnosis, and these symptoms cause severe impairment in a person's life. The prognosis, of course, is going to be worse for the severe forms of the disorder.

ADHD is a serious condition that usually doesn't vanish completely in adulthood, although in some cases, symptoms will diminish. Perhaps the discussion above will help you feel more reassured about your child's future. On the other hand, it may point out areas that need some work.

PART II

The Diagnosis of ADHD

CHAPTER 6
Getting the Right Information

CHAPTER 7
Putting the Data Together

6

GETTING THE RIGHT
INFORMATION

A DIAGNOSTIC EVALUATION FOR ADHD needs to be done very carefully, and it generally takes about four hours of office time. What we're looking for is the following in someone's life:

a. A pattern of inattention and/or hyperactivity/impulsivity
b. Persistence of this pattern for at least six months
c. Behavior inconsistent with developmental level
d. Symptoms that significantly interfere with home, school, or work functioning

However, the diagnosis of attention-deficit/hyperactivity disorder can be tricky. First, there is no specific test for ADHD. An ADHD evaluation is different from diagnosis in physical medicine, or even from diagnosis with other types of psychological difficulties. There is no one physical, neurological, or psychological test that can prove or disprove the existence of ADHD. It would certainly come in handy if there were!

The second reason why diagnosing ADHD is tricky is that, oddly enough, the face-to-face interview with the child in the office is often one of the least helpful parts of the evaluation process. Research has shown that *80 percent of children with ADHD will sit still in a doctor's office*—no matter how they behave the rest of the time.[1] Why? Because the situation is usually fairly intimidating to a child, it may be somewhat new or interesting as well, and sometimes, it is one-on-one. I can think of many instances in which frustrated parents have told a doctor or mental health professional how difficult and impossible their child's behavior was, only to have the doctor or professional dismiss the possibility of ADHD simply because the child sat still in the office.

The third reason is that many children with ADHD cannot accurately recall or describe their past experiences. Other children with ADHD can recall past events well enough, but they are defensive, unwilling to admit any problems, and many kids with ADHD put an overly favorable spin on their descriptions of their academic and social lives.

The result is that the diagnostic process must involve a lot of information collecting from multiple sources in addition to the child's testimony. The child must be seen by a health professional, but what is primarily needed is detailed information about the child's school, home, and social functioning. This information should include a careful developmental history, as well as a thorough description of the parents' primary concerns. Information about a child should be gathered from many sources, including parents and teachers.

Who can competently conduct an evaluation for attention-deficit/ hyperactivity disorder? Any mental health professional or physician *trained and experienced in the evaluation of ADHD.* A pediatrician could do the diagnosis if he or she had the proper amount of time as well as expertise, and so could a psychiatric social worker or psychologist. A physician is not necessary for the diagnosis of ADHD, although a physician's involvement does become necessary if medication is being considered.

The Diagnostic Process

The evaluation for ADHD should involve the following steps. The goal of the evaluation is to determine if ADHD exists, and if it does, to plan for treatment and to educate and prepare the family for that process.

Before the First Meeting with Parents

After a family has called for an appointment, many clinicians send a packet of questionnaires and evaluation forms to parents and teachers. After these forms are filled out, the family can be scheduled for the initial meeting. The packet that goes to the family (usually the parents) includes items such as instructions, family information, medical history, developmental history, a general child psychopathology rating form (e.g., Achenbach's Child Behavior Checklist, 2001), an ADHD rating scale, and Barkley's Home Situations Questionnaire (Barkley & Murphy, 2006).

After a release of information has been signed, the child's teachers receive a packet containing the teacher version of the Child Behavior Checklist, Barkley's School Situations Questionnaire, a teacher version of an ADHD rating scale, and some kind of social skills evaluation instrument.

The Parent Interview

Next is an interview with the parents to cover the presenting problems, developmental history, and family history, and to plan the rest of the evaluation procedures. The parents' presenting concerns should be compared to the *DSM-5* criteria for ADHD, the other ADHD characteristics mentioned in chapter 1. The clinician should also compare presenting complaints to the *DSM-5* criteria for possible comorbid conditions, such as ODD, CD, depression, and anxiety.

A number of structured interview formats are available to help accomplish the objectives mentioned above. Barkley's Clinical Interview–Parent Report Form (from *Defiant Children, Second Edition: A Clinician's Manual for Assessment and Parent Training*) is useful in this regard. This form covers ODD and CD symptoms before getting to ADHD, to give parents a chance to "simmer down" before talking about the possibility of attention-deficit/hyperactivity disorder.

The Diagnostic Interview Schedule for Children (DISC) is also popular with mental health professionals. All childhood disorders in the *DSM-5* are included. To speed up the interview process, key features of each disorder are inquired about first. If the key features are not there, the interviewer then flips to the next diagnosis.

The child's parents are the most vital source of information. They should be taken very seriously and approached with a nonjudgmental attitude. The evaluator must keep in mind that, if the child has ADHD, the cause is not faulty parenting but rather an inherited condition. There are several reasons why it isn't always easy to remember this. First, many parents are so stressed by their child's behavior that they do not exactly make the best impression on the diagnostician. They can come across as angry, hysterical, depressed, or worse, and therapists with a strong leaning toward family dynamic theory will often conclude, "No wonder the kid is having such a rough time—I'd be hyperactive myself with parents like these!" Many parents, however, will accurately report that they were not so emotionally disturbed— and even considered themselves fairly normal—before their child arrived on the scene.

Second, there is evidence that the biological parents of children with ADHD show a higher incidence of certain other psychological problems. These problems can include alcoholism (and/or drug abuse), depression, sociopathy, anxiety, and, of course, ADHD itself. Many parents also have more than one of these difficulties, which can make the diagnostician's job of relating to them even more challenging.

Third, there is a higher incidence of marital dissatisfaction, separation, and divorce in families where there is a child with ADHD, so the couple may disagree and argue during the interview about the child, as well as about other issues. If only one parent is able or willing to come to the session, he or she may show the effects of the stress resulting from living with not only one but two people with ADHD—the child and the spouse.

The first topic covered with parents is what brings them to the office. A general question about presenting problems should be asked initially and then, if ADHD is suspected, more specific inquiries into other possible symptoms/problems that may not have been spontaneously mentioned, such as emotional overarousal, difficulty delaying gratification, or disorganization. When ADHD-C is involved, the presenting problems that parents mention usually focus on issues such as school underachievement, domestic difficulties in living with the child, social problems, and other kinds of disruptive behavior. With ADHD-PI, however, problems are not as much "in your face," and parents are often more bewildered. Their complaints focus more on disorganization, amazing forgetfulness, inability to finish things, and general "spaciness."

Following a detailed analysis of the presenting problems, a developmental history should be taken. A number of structured developmental history forms are available. When an ADHD screening is being done, this history should involve more than just the usual developmental milestones, such as when the child walked and talked. Since many experts feel that ADHD symptoms can appear in 60 to 70 percent of kids who will eventually be diagnosed around the age of three (usually ADHD-C), the interviewer should specifically inquire about the development of the ADHD symptoms listed previously, such as impulsivity, hyperactivity, impatience, emotional overarousal, noncompliance, and social aggressiveness.[2]

Information about pregnancy, labor, and delivery are also relevant, since there is a possibility that, in some situations, prenatal, perinatal, or postnatal injury to the brain may produce ADHD or something akin to it. Low birth weight is also frequently associated with later diagnosis of ADHD.

Infant characteristics are not reliable predictors of the disorder, but there are significant mild correlations between ADHD and infant temperaments involving negative responses to change or new situations, more time spent in a negative mood (including colic), and exaggerated emotional responsiveness. After three to six months of age, the list of ADHD infancy correlates can include resistance to cuddling, high activity level, sleep and feeding disturbances, and monotonous, ongoing vocalizations or crying. Keep in mind, however, that these are not definitive signs. A lot of difficult babies turn out not to have ADHD.

After taking the developmental history, a family history should be explored due to the hereditary nature of ADHD. The father is usually "picked on" first with a question such as "How did you do in elementary school?" The focus here is often limited to things like concentration, grades, and misbehavior, because it is difficult for people to remember that far back. The mother is then asked similar questions to explore the possibility that Mom had ADHD-PI. Health care professionals should explain to parents why these questions are being asked, because this is often the first time many parents have heard the notion that their child's problems may be hereditary. Next, inquiries about other relatives, including siblings, are often helpful. The interviewer is looking for signs of childhood or adult ADHD symptoms, as well as signs of depression, substance abuse, anxiety, and antisocial personality.

Finally, the initial parent interview should conclude with cooperative planning of the rest of the evaluation, and, if ADHD is suspected, some way for the parents to learn more about this disorder (seminars, books, videos, support group meetings, etc.). This educational component is an extremely helpful part of the diagnostic process. Many parents will almost be able to make the diagnosis themselves after hearing more about the common problems and typical developmental course of untreated ADHD. In addition, many of the fathers—and some of the mothers—will recognize themselves in the descriptions. This awareness may lead to the possibility of their being treated for adult ADHD, which, of course, will prove immensely valuable to the management of their child's problems.

Education about ADHD should be done only if ADHD is strongly suspected after talking with the parents and reviewing the results of the rating scales. The evaluator should also inform the parents about the possibility of ADHD look-alikes, as well as comorbid disorders. It is helpful to keep in mind that the factors that often discriminate ADHD-C from other disorders are early onset, nature of symptoms (inattention and hyperactivity/impulsivity), and consistent, chronic course.

The Child Interview

The interview with the child comes next in the diagnostic process. The goal of interviewing the child is to rule out more serious disorders, such as psychosis, to see how willing the child is to talk, to get as much information as possible about how the child perceives his school, home, and social life, and to begin to build a good relationship between the child and the diagnostician or therapist, which may be necessary for later work.

As mentioned before, when interviewing the child for the first time, *the diagnostician will probably not see hyperactive or impulsive symptoms in the office.* There certainly are some young children who cannot sit still and who will be in constant motion and/or constantly chatty. These children will appear only about 20 percent of the time, and they are much more likely to have ADHD.

One good way to begin the session with a child is to say in a matter-of-fact way something like, "I assume it wasn't your idea to come here." This tactic is especially good for older children and teens. Most kids do not want to see any doctor, and this statement lets them know it's not unusual to feel that way. This introduction often helps the child talk more freely. Most children will talk, although with widely varying degrees of accuracy and truthfulness. It is important that the interviewer not try to be too friendly. Children will frequently become suspicious of an adult who seems too syrupy or condescending.

Older children can sit and talk for forty-five minutes to an hour, and many will open up quite a bit when talking with an adult who is sincerely trying to understand them. Many of these children are so used to being criticized that being treated with respect is a refreshing experience for them. With smaller children, having them draw or play while they talk is often useful, although the session may still have to be kept shorter, perhaps limited to half an hour.

When a child is too defensive to be able to tolerate sitting and talking about problems, several options are possible. One is to begin by talking about enjoyable topics or strengths. One little boy warmed up considerably while discussing fireworks. Some children are actually quite interested in the school information collected, such as their old report cards or achievement test scores. These items can often be discussed fruitfully.

Toward the end of the session, the child is told just what the rest of the evaluation process will involve, and older children may be given some say in the design of that process. Some children, for example, don't like the idea of school questionnaires, because they don't want anyone at their school knowing they are seeing a "shrink." Reassurance about confidentiality may be in order. Other children may be interested in doing psychological testing if they think it might reveal some of their strengths.

There are a number of child self-report forms available that children can fill out (if they are old enough), and these can later be used in a semistructured interview format. Children with ADHD-C usually underreport their own disruptive (externalizing) behavior, so parents and teachers are better sources in that regard.[3] Parents and teachers, on the other hand, often miss childhood symptoms of anxiety and depression (internalizing disorders), which children themselves can often report more accurately.[4]

Other Rating Scales

Rating scales are often referred to as either broad-band or narrow-band. Broad-band scales, like the Child Behavior Checklist (CBCL) or Behavior Assessment System for Children-3 (BASC-3), cover a wide range of possible problems. They provide a kind of overview of a child's functioning. The CBCL, for example, offers parent, teacher, and child versions, and it has a number of subscales:

a.   aggressive behavior
b.   delinquent behavior
c.   anxious/depressed
d.   somatic complaints
e.   social problems
f.   attention problems
g.   thought problems
h.   withdrawn social skills

Narrow-band scales are used when the evaluator wants to look more closely at a potential problem area, such as a possible comorbid condition or even an alternative diagnosis. Narrow-band scales are usually used when a diagnostic question pops up during the course of the overall evaluation. These rating scales include instruments for the following: depression, anxiety, obsessive compulsive disorder (OCD), and Tourette's syndrome.

School Information

The collection of information (present and past) from school, such as grades, teacher observations, achievement test scores, and current placement, is time consuming but very important. ADHD is a condition that starts early in life, so most children with ADHD will have had problems with school for a long time. Preschool problems are usually behavioral. Primary grade problems often involve both behavioral (hyperactive/impulsive) and academic (inattentive) concerns.

A priority is collecting previous grades—and actual report cards if possible—all the way back to kindergarten. Many parents save report cards, and they are helpful not only for the grades themselves, but also for the teachers' comments. With children who may have ADHD, comments related to the basic symptoms are frequent and reappear year after year. These persistent observations can include "always wandering around," "bothers others," "blurts out answers," "too easily gotten off task," and so on.

The grades of a child with ADHD can be extremely variable. Middle-school children with ADHD (grades six through eight), for example, will often get one of every possible grade, from A to F, on the same report card. This variability is due to the teacher and subject-sensitivity of the child, who can often function well if she likes the teacher and the subject, but who can go the opposite direction if she doesn't. It is also not unusual for grades to vary tremendously for the same subject for the four quarters of the school year. But since underachievement is the hallmark of the child with ADHD, the child's grades will usually not match her ability level.

Achievement test scores are also gathered, going back in time as far as possible. The interpretation of these can be somewhat difficult. Achievement tests are group administered, and children with ADHD usually do more poorly in a group than in a one-to-one situation. With many of these children, therefore, the achievement test scores will often not measure up to overall ability. If the child can remember taking these tests, it is helpful to ask her if she recalls really trying hard to do her best, or if she blew the tests off by impulsively guessing or by making patterns on the computer answer sheets.

On the other hand, some children produce achievement test scores that are *better* than the child's grades for the same subjects. This unusual finding is reassuring, and the reasons for the discrepancy should be carefully explained to both parents and child. Achievement test scores that are better than the child's grades may indicate that *the child is learning the material*, even though the child's grades are not good. Both parents and child will be glad to hear this!

The achievement scores are more useful for clinical information than for determining the existence of attention-deficit/hyperactivity disorder. Since there are many more ways to artificially lower test scores (illness, bad mood, distractibility) than there are to artificially raise them (cheating), a fairly safe assumption is to take the achievement scores to be a *minimum* estimate of the child's actual achievement—and perhaps of her ability as well.

As part of the evaluation, the child's current placement in school should also be noted. If the child is in special education, psychological testing and staffing reports are collected. Once the evaluator has gotten the school information listed above, a phone call to the teacher (or teachers) is in order. Talking to the child's teacher is invaluable. The conversation provides three critical bits of data: (1) reliable information about the child's school functioning, (2) an idea of how the teacher feels about this student, and (3) some idea of how the teacher feels about ADHD. The last item often has important implications for later treatment.

7
PUTTING THE DATA TOGETHER

SINCE THERE IS NO one definitive diagnostic procedure or test for ADHD, the final determination of whether a child qualifies for this diagnosis must rely on an integration of all the data collected. The following questions help make sense out of that mass of information. In addition to making a statement, it is important to also describe a profile of strengths for this particular child.

Integration of the Data

Question 1: Does the child qualify for six or more out of the nine items on one or both of the *DSM-5* symptom lists for inattention and for hyperactivity/impulsivity?

Inattention

 a. fails to pay close attention to details or makes careless mistakes
 b. has difficulty sustaining attention in work or play
 c. does not listen when spoken to directly

d.   fails to finish schoolwork, chores, or work duties

e.   has difficulty organizing activities

f.   avoids tasks requiring sustained mental effort

g.   loses things

h.   is easily distracted

i.   is forgetful

Hyperactivity/Impulsivity

Hyperactivity

a.   fidgets or squirms in seat

b.   leaves seat when remaining seated is expected

c.   runs about or climbs in situations where this is inappropriate

d.   has difficulty playing quietly

e.   acts as if "driven by a motor"

f.   talks excessively

Impulsivity

a.   blurts out answers before the question is completed

b.   has difficulty awaiting turn

c.   interrupts or intrudes on others

Do the presenting complaints show a pattern that is persistent and which started early in life? Are the frequency and severity of the symptoms such that they are extraordinary even for the age of the child, cause significant impairment in the child's life, and cause trouble in two or more settings?

I also like to match the presenting problems with the eight ADHD characteristics listed in chapter 1. Although this list overlaps to some extent with the *DSM-5* list, it also includes items that are a little different but which many parents can relate to easily. These items include difficulty delaying gratification, emotional overarousal, noncompliance, and social difficulties. Comparison of this eight-item list to the child's experiences is a good way of evaluating impairment.

Question 2: Another good indicator of actual impairment (and not just abstract symptoms) is this: how does the developmental history taken from the parents match the typical course of untreated ADHD-C or ADHD-PI (chapter 3)? Answering this question involves looking for the manifestations of the symptoms listed above but also being aware of how the picture changes with age. Early hyperactivity, for example, will simmer down quite a bit by adolescence. Inattentive kids do not show many problems until they hit the primary grades. Retention in school is common in the early years but has been known to occur with some children diagnosed with ADHD as late as middle school.

Question 3: Who else in the family has ADHD and/or the other conditions that often accompany ADHD? An important indicator here is what we often call the chip-off-the-old-block syndrome. A father may say, for example, that when he was in elementary school, his performance and behavior were very similar to his son's. If this observation is offered without much doubt or hesitation, we often consider it evidence for genetic transmission. If a child has ADHD, the chance that one or both parents also have ADHD is 40 to 50 percent. A previously diagnosed sibling is also a red flag and raises the chances of ADHD in the child being evaluated from about 5 percent to about 30 percent.

Question 4: Is the information from the child consistent with ADHD symptoms? Some children with ADHD can and do describe typical symptoms in their own words. Those problems most often described accurately include distractibility, boredom, and sometimes emotional intensity. Other ADHD traits may not be mentioned because the child sees them as weaknesses, such as hyperactivity or problems getting along with other children.

Other children reveal symptoms verbally but indirectly, saying they hate school "because of the work" or consistently blaming other people—teachers, playmates, parents—for whatever problems they have. Some children who may have ADHD will show hyperactive and impulsive kinds of behavior in the classroom, such as fidgeting, walking or running around, speaking rapidly and loudly, interrupting, and being distracted by the various objects in the room. As mentioned earlier, these children have a higher probability of having ADHD.

Question 5: Does the child score above the cutoffs for ADHD on the structured rating scales? Are more than 50 percent of the situations checked as problems on the Home and School Situations Questionnaires? How severe are the ratings?

Question 6: Does the school and achievement testing information support the notion that the child is not working to capacity? To what extent might learning disabilities account for this underachievement if it exists?

Question 7: Do the parents—after becoming more familiar with ADHD through an educational seminar, book, video, or online information—feel that their child could have ADHD? Many of the parents who say "That's my kid!" are correct. Remember that parents have many more images and recollections about their child than they could ever share with any diagnostician in three or four hours. When parents encounter two hours or more of an educational program about ADHD, they can match more of their many thoughts and memories with the program.

Two cautions are important here. First, the fact that true ADHD is not caused by faulty parenting is an appealing idea to parents, and it may bias their perceptions. Second, the possibility of comorbidity and ADHD look-alikes must be kept in mind.

Comorbidity and ADHD Look-Alikes

Recent research on ADHD has confirmed and clarified what we have suspected for some time: ADHD is often accompanied by other psychological problems.[1] These other diagnoses will fall under the categories of disruptive disorders, anxiety disorders, mood disorders, and learning disabilities. A minority of children with ADHD will have what is sometimes called "pure" or "squeaky-clean" ADHD: they will have an ADHD diagnosis and nothing else.

Below are listed the possible comorbid disorders and the approximate percentage of children with ADHD who will show that problem (whether it's diagnosed or not) by their midadolescent years.

Most of these comorbid disorders are to some extent ADHD look-alikes. They share common characteristics with ADHD, and consequently, they can sometimes be mistaken for ADHD. After all, concentration impairments can accompany many childhood psychological problems, including depression and anxiety. Disruptive behavior, on the other hand, is central to ADHD, ODD, and CD. It is therefore important to keep in mind the different diagnostic possibilities:

> ## Key Concept
> ADHD is often accompanied by other psychological diagnoses, including disruptive disorders, anxiety disorders, mood disorders, and learning disabilities.

1. ADHD exists by itself.
2. Another disorder exists by itself (without ADHD).
3. Two (or more) disorders exist together.
4. No disorder exists.

Oppositional Defiant Disorder

(50–60 percent):[2] ADHD and ODD show a tremendous amount of overlap. Children with ADHD can be obnoxious due to their hyperactivity and impulsivity, but they don't usually mean to irritate you. Children with ODD, on the other hand, have their primary problem with authority. They are negative, defiant, resistive, and deliberately (not so much forgetfully or impulsively) disobedient. Like children with ADHD, kids with ODD have bad tempers, argue, and blame others for their own mistakes. Unlike kids with ADHD, though, children with ODD are spiteful, vindictive, and purposely try to irritate other people. Symptoms of ODD usually start at home, then may also move to school. Unlike children with ADHD, children who just have ODD are able to focus appropriately, complete schoolwork, and show few behavior problems in the early grades.

Conduct Disorder

(30–40 percent):[3] CD may be the modern euphemism for juvenile delinquency. Children with ADHD don't want to irritate you, but sometimes they do. Children with ODD do want to irritate you, and they become very good at it. Children with CD want to hurt you or others. They don't care if they make you angry, and they are more aggressive than children with ODD. Children with CD threaten, bully, and fight. They can be physically cruel to people as well as animals. Children with CD steal, force others into sexual activity, set fires, and destroy property. They frequently break rules by staying out too late, running away, or skipping school.

Children with ODD often "graduate" to CD as the years pass. This graduation is more likely if they have comorbid ADHD, and if they come from disruptive, unstable families. Children with CD generally are not good treatment candidates. Ironically, I have found that they are better treatment candidates if their CD isn't their only problem. If their difficult behavior is also related to another disorder that is more treatable, such as ADHD, depression, or bipolar illness, the prognosis is better. This is one of the few occasions where comorbidity can be a plus!

Anxiety Disorders

(30 percent):[4] Boys and girls with ADHD show a strong tendency toward anxiety problems, and when they do have such a problem, these kids often have *more than one anxiety disorder.*[5] In addition to ADHD, for example, they might show two of the following: separation anxiety, generalized anxiety disorder, and obsessive-compulsive disorder (OCD). Social phobia and panic attacks may develop in older children. The characteristic of emotional overarousal, mentioned earlier, can certainly affect the child's experience of anxiety as well as anger.

On the other hand, there is some evidence that comorbid anxiety may have a moderating effect on ADHD impulsivity. People with social anxiety, for example, often hold back because they obsess about making mistakes and looking stupid in front of others. That is the opposite of impulsivity.

Major Depression

(20–30 percent):[6] An episode of major depression is characterized primarily by a period of two weeks or more in which an individual shows a depressed mood and/or a drastically reduced interest in just about everything. This episode must be a major alteration in the person's usual way of functioning; it involves symptoms such as a change in weight, fatigue, restlessness, increased or decreased sleeping, feelings of worthlessness, poor concentration, and thoughts of death. In children and adolescents, the depressed mood may show itself primarily as irritability.

Disruptive Mood Dysregulation Disorder

Related to bipolar disorder is the new *DSM-5* diagnosis of disruptive mood dysregulation disorder (DMDD). DMDD includes children who have severe verbal or physical temper tantrums three or more times per week. The tantrums are way out of proportion to the events that trigger them, developmentally inappropriate, and the child's mood in between tantrums is consistently irritable or angry. DMDD in some (but not all) ways overlaps with the symptom of emotional overarousal mentioned earlier. At this time, the relationship between ADHD and DMDD is uncertain.[7]

Tic Disorders

(10 percent):[8] Tics are sudden, short-lived, and repetitive motor movements (eye blinking, shoulder shrugging, facial grimaces) or vocalizations (throat clearing, grunting, sniffing). Tics can occur in complex forms, such as repeating phrases or engaging in repetitive grooming behavior. These impulses are usually experienced as irresistible, although sometimes a person can temporarily suppress them. They also happen less during sleep. When tics do occur, they are usually only mild to moderate in severity. Tic symptoms usually diminish—and sometimes disappear entirely—during adolescence and adulthood.

When both motor and vocal tics have been going on for some time and produce marked distress, Tourette's syndrome may be diagnosed. While only a small percentage of children with ADHD will also have Tourette's, it has been estimated that 60 percent of children with Tourette's also qualify as ADHD.[9] Differential diagnosis here is important, because it has implications for medication treatment. Recently, with increased media exposure in popular culture and support groups, tic disorders have become more well-known and understood, but they may also have become more feared. It is important to keep in mind that tic disorders are rarely incapacitating, and when they coexist with ADHD, the ADHD is most often the more serious problem.

Sleep Disorders

(30–50 percent):[10] Most parents of children with ADHD are very aware of the fact that their children are not good sleepers. As these children become older, getting them up in the morning also becomes harder and harder, because they didn't go to bed in time to get enough sleep. But it's also true that children and adults with ADHD take longer to get to sleep and wake more frequently during the night.[11] As a matter of fact, a number of years ago, one theory had it that ADHD was caused by sleep deprivation.[12] Although this belief is not accurate, sleep deprivation may have a significant impact not only on ADHD but also on comorbid disorders such as anxiety and depression.

Learning Disabilities

(35 percent):[13] Distinguishing between ADHD and LD is a difficult—and not always possible—task to accomplish. The two categories often overlap. Perhaps 35 percent of kids with ADHD will have a learning disability, and 25 percent of children with LD may have ADHD. And many children have one challenge and not the other.

Learning disabilities that often accompany ADHD include reading problems (dyslexia), difficulty with math computation and story problems, strong aversions to handwritten assignments, and what are sometimes called nonverbal learning disabilities. LD problems cause achievement in one or more academic areas that is much lower than what would be expected based on intellectual ability. Learning disabilities are chronic, invisible (like ADHD), and unrelated to IQ.

There are several ways to distinguish attention deficit from learning disability.

The first is the developmental history. Most children with LD only will not show at age two or three the ADHD symptoms of hyperactivity, impulsivity, emotional overarousal, social aggressiveness, and so on. Some children with LD only, though, may show these behaviors after years and years of academic frustration.

Second, if the child's IQ and achievement test scores are not discrepant and are considered valid, LD may be ruled out by definition.

Third, if from the early school years on, there are consistent comments about distractibility itself and short attention span, one leans toward ADHD as the diagnosis. Children with LD only are more prone to looking distractible when working on tasks that involve their weak areas; on other tasks, their attention may be normal.

Finally, a medication trial will often eliminate a lot of ADHD symptoms. If a medicated child is able to function fairly normally in an academic setting and no longer underachieves, it would appear that the problem was ADHD alone. Few people believe that medication will help with a true learning disability.

Idiosyncratic Patterns

Several factors can make substantial changes in the typical ADHD symptom picture and may, consequently, cause a diagnosis to be missed in a child that genuinely has ADHD. These factors include the following:

1. **Good social skills.** A significant number of children with ADHD—even combined types—get along well with their peers. These kids have friends, are not overly bossy, and may not show the usual low frustration tolerance in competitive situations. In some of these children, some of the ADHD symptoms are moderated just enough to become social assets. Bossiness, for example, may become leadership, or excessive energy may make the child "the life of the party."

2. **High IQ.** Children with ADHD can not only succeed in school but may also actually enjoy it. Because of their academic success and the reinforcement they receive from parents and teachers, very bright kids may *inhibit* inappropriate behavior while at school. However, many of these youngsters will go off like rockets when they come home, and their ADHD symptoms then make family life miserable for the rest of the evening. This kind of behavior pattern often leads evaluators to conclude incorrectly that the parents or the family itself is the problem.

3. **Shyness.** From the earlier descriptions of children with ADHD (especially ADHD-C), these kids sound anything but shy. Instead, they seem indifferent about how others see them, and they come across as socially boorish. We now know, though, that about 30 percent of these children will also experience anxiety problems.[14] Some kids with ADHD are extremely concerned about the opinions of others. In public, these children inhibit their hyperactive/impulsive behavior, but—like the high IQ child—they usually show their ADHD symptoms at home. In some of these children, shyness has been aggravated by difficulties with coordination, speech, learning disabilities, or ADHD-PI itself that made these kids targets of ridicule from peers.

4. **No siblings, or one-on-one preschool situation with parents.** In some children, problems do not appear until the child reaches the primary grades. These kids may have ADHD-PI. Others, however, show a developmental history that seems to lack parental reports of extreme hyperactivity, impulsivity, emotional overarousal, and so on during the child's preschool years. Sometimes, the reason for this apparent absence of symptoms is the lack of siblings at home during these years; the youngster may have been an only child, or perhaps the siblings were either much older or were not born yet. *Lack of sibling rivalry and a one-on-one (or one-on-two) situation with parents can moderate ADHD symptoms considerably.*

The lack of competition, in addition to having reasonably competent and attentive parents, can produce fairly normal behavior, at least for a while.

5. **Inattentive presentation.** ADHD without hyperactivity is still overlooked too frequently. When hyperactivity is not a problem in the early years, other possible ADHD characteristics, such as emotional overarousal and social aggressiveness, are also moderated or are nonexistent. In this case, the diagnostic evaluation must focus heavily on the existence of characteristics such as major concentration difficulties, disorganization, forgetfulness, passive noncompliance, and inability to finish things. Inattentive children may not be disruptive, but they are still unsuccessful, and they are still suffering.

The Post-Diagnostic Interview

Once all the information has been collected, the child and parents have been interviewed, and the evaluation has been completed, it's time to explain the results to everyone. Many children with ADHD, of course, are not very interested in talking about something called ADHD, but it's important to try to explain the problem (*their* particular version of ADHD) and the treatment to kids as best one can. These days, there are a number of books for children that describe ADHD from a child's point of view.

Parents, however, are *very* interested in hearing what the problem is. Clinicians must keep in mind that most parents have been "educated" about ADHD through the Internet, newspapers, magazines, and television. ADHD is a household word, and parents may think they know a lot about it. Parents' store of knowledge, however, may include a lot of good—as well as a lot of inaccurate—information. Before trying to explain the problem and its treatment, therefore, it is helpful if the therapist firsts asks what the parents (and the child) have already heard about ADHD. One young boy, for example, was mixing up ADHD and AIDS. The evaluator must listen carefully and sympathetically to whatever is said before attempting to correct or reinforce any piece of information.

The post-diagnostic interview is also the time to prepare the parents and child—and to motivate them—for the treatment plan. A number of issues need to be understood from the beginning. ADHD, for example, is a chronic problem that is not outgrown. Treatment, therefore, also needs to be ongoing. You don't necessarily need to come in weekly for the rest of your life, but you also shouldn't stop entirely. Continuing education for parents and children about ADHD is critical. Mom and Dad might consider joining a support group. Medication and treatment need to be explained over and over. Drug treatment, for example, is actually very safe and very effective, but it can sometimes take a while to find the right medication for a particular child. Other issues such as social skills and educational underachievement may need to be addressed.

The post-diagnostic interview lays the groundwork for the future. With good treatment, parents and children may be able to look forward to reasonable success and happiness. With poor or no treatment, the coming years can bring increasing failure and dissatisfaction.

8

EDUCATION ABOUT ADHD
AND COUNSELING

ONCE THE DIAGNOSTIC EVALUATION has been completed and parents learn of their child's ADHD diagnosis, there are a lot of things parents need to understand and a lot of things parents will need to do during the years your children are growing up. It's quite a job, but it can be done! Especially if you get the right kind of assistance.

First of all, there's a ton of information about ADHD that you'll need to learn. This book is a great start. You can also get good information from CHADD.org and ADD.org, the websites of Children and Adults with Attention Deficit Disorder and the Attention Deficit Disorder Association, respectively. While these are reputable websites with good information, be careful of the Internet, TV, and magazine information. It's too often distorted, sensational, or just plain wrong. Look at the table of contents of this book. That's the stuff you'll have to master in order to best raise your child with ADHD.

Educating parents about ADHD is the most important part of any ADHD treatment plan.

Second, once you become better informed about ADHD, you're going to want to apply your newfound knowledge toward working with health care professionals to design your child's treatment plan. This plan will include important decisions about the following:

1. Explaining ADHD to family and friends.
2. The kind of counseling/follow-up/monitoring that will be necessary for the child.
3. The kind of counseling/follow-up/monitoring that will be necessary for parents and guardians.
4. What self-control or social skills training will be needed for the child.
5. The approach that will be taken to behavior management at home.
6. The way medication treatment will be handled.
7. The kinds of adjustments or accommodations that will be needed at the school.

Third, designing a treatment plan will involve examining many of your own personal (and often strong!) thoughts and feelings about issues like child discipline, medication, friends, self-control, ADHD itself, teaching, family values, and even your own personality. If you have a spouse or a former spouse or partner, their thoughts and feelings about these same issues will also come into play.

Fourth, except in rare cases, all the thoughts and feelings and people just mentioned will be too much to deal with without professional assistance. You'll need to find a friendly mental health professional who's knowledgeable about ADHD to meet with you over the years. This person will help you sort out your reactions and attitudes so you will not only make a good treatment plan but also follow it.

It will be a good idea to see this counselor periodically during the time your child is growing up with you. The counselor may also see your son or daughter who has ADHD. Don't worry—this doesn't necessarily mean weekly visits for the next fifteen years! A more plausible plan is to do the ADHD evaluation (three to four visits), then three months or so of weekly sessions to get the situation stabilized, then phase down the session frequency to as low as once or twice a year. But stay in touch! That way, you can always increase the frequency of sessions temporarily as special problems arise. Rest assured that when you live with a child with ADHD, life is going to throw plenty of curveballs at you. You are going to regularly need expert moral support you can count on.

Your Treatment Goals

What will you be trying to accomplish with all your efforts to learn about ADHD and make a solid treatment plan? Your first goal is for children with ADHD to be able to get rid of their parents! You want them to grow up, leave home, become financially independent, and maybe start a family of their own. Your second goal is for your child to enjoy their growing-up years with you and for you to enjoy them too. Your third goal is to prevent ADHD comorbidities: oppositional defiance and conduct disorder (mostly for ADHD-C) and anxiety and depression (mostly for ADHD-PI). Your final goal is to enjoy yourself and your spouse or partner (if applicable) as much as possible *separate from your child with ADHD*. It is a big mistake to eat, sleep, and drink ADHD; doing so will make you absolutely no fun to be with.

> **Key Concept**
> Your first goal is for children with ADHD to be able to get rid of their parents! You want them to grow up, leave home, become financially independent, and maybe start a family of their own.

What's Your ADHD IQ?

So educating yourself as a parent about ADHD is critical. Here's our twenty-question ADHD multiple choice test (followed by the answers). Let's see how much you've learned so far. Then, in the last part of this chapter, we'll look at the role of counseling in the treatment of ADHD.

Twenty-Question ADHD Multiple Choice Test

See how many questions you can answer correctly on our ADHD multiple choice test (MCT). Be careful, because some items may have more than one correct answer, or they may have no correct answers at all. Our ADHD MCT is tough—but so is raising a child with the disorder! The correct answers are provided in the section following the test.

1. ADHD-C refers to:
    a. the complex presentation of ADHD
    b. the chronic presentation of ADHD
    c. the combined presentation of ADHD
    d. the critical presentation of ADHD

2. ADHD-PI refers to:
    a. the predominantly insidious presentation of ADHD
    b. the predominantly inattentive presentation of ADHD
    c. the predominantly intelligent presentation of ADHD
    d. the predominantly invisible presentation of ADHD

3. As a child with ADHD grows older and matures, his symptom of hyperactivity *usually* will:
    a. get worse
    b. get better
    c. disappear
    d. stay the same

4. ADHD can often be diagnosed when the child is as young as:
    a. adolescence
    b. first grade
    c. junior high
    d. the preschool years

5. The most useful test for ADHD is:
    a. a genetic blood test

    b. an EEG

    c. a urinalysis

    d. the Wechsler IQ test

6.   ADHD can be diagnosed by a:

    a. neurologist

    b. psychologist

    c. physician

    d. mental health professional

7.   An ADHD evaluation should take approximately:

    a. fifteen minutes if the child is hyperactive

    b. one hour under most circumstances

    c. three to four hours

    d. ten hours or more

8.   In a doctor's office, the child with ADHD will usually:

    a. show his ADHD symptoms quickly

    b. sit still

    c. not leave his mother's side

    d. tear the place apart

9.   Children with ADHD usually respond better to their:

    a. fathers than to their mothers

    b. mothers than to their fathers

    c. babysitters than to their teachers

    d. none of the above

10. Research has shown that ADHD is primarily:

    a. learned or acquired as the child grows up

    b. hereditary

    c. caused by ineffective parenting

    d. caused by diet

11. If a child has a sibling who has ADHD, that child's chances
    of also having ADHD are:
    a. zero
    b. 100 percent
    c. 70 percent
    d. 30 percent

12. Which is *not* a useful prognostic indicator with ADHD?
    a. socioeconomic status
    b. hobbies
    c. intelligence
    d. social skills

13. Which is a possible cause of ADHD in some kids?
    a. poor sleep
    b. sugar
    c. allergies
    d. lead

14. Kids with ADHD can often sit and concentrate in situations
    that are:
    a. novel
    b. interesting
    c. intimidating
    d. one-on-one

15. Impulsivity refers to:
    a. thinking without acting
    b. acting and carefully thinking
    c. postponing action
    d. acting without thinking

16. With peers, kids with ADHD often tend to be:
    a. indifferent
    b. intrusive

    c. too placid

    d. too cooperative

17. Externalizing disorders:
    a. don't bother anyone
    b. bother oneself but not others
    c. bother others but not oneself
    d. bother only parents

18. Another way of looking at ADHD is to see it as:
    a. a problem with self-abuse
    b. a problem with self-control
    c. a problem with thinking straight
    d. a problem with depression

19. What percentage of kids with ADHD will sit still in a doctor's office?
    a. 10 percent
    b. 40 percent
    c. 80 percent
    d. 95 percent

20. A developmental history is critical to diagnosis and should be carefully taken from:
    a. the child
    b. the teacher
    c. close relatives from outside the family
    d. the parents

Answer Key

The correct answer(s) to each question are in bold.

1. ADHD-C refers to:
    a. the complex presentation of ADHD

   b. the chronic presentation of ADHD

   c. **the combined presentation of ADHD**

   d. the critical presentation of ADHD

2.   ADHD-PI refers to:

   a. the predominantly insidious presentation of ADHD

   b. **the predominantly inattentive presentation of ADHD**

   c. the predominantly intelligent presentation of ADHD

   d. the predominantly invisible presentation of ADHD

3.   As a child with ADHD grows older and matures, his symptom of hyperactivity *usually* will:

   a. get worse

   b. **get better**

   c. disappear

   d. stay the same

4.   ADHD can often be diagnosed when the child is as young as:

   a. adolescence

   b. first grade

   c. junior high

   d. **the preschool years**

5.   The most useful test for ADHD is:

   a. a genetic blood test

   b. an EEG

   c. a urinalysis

   d. the Wechsler IQ test

There is no correct answer here! ADHD cannot be diagnosed by a single test.

6.   ADHD can be diagnosed by a:

   a. **neurologist**

b. **psychologist**

c. **physician**

d. **mental health professional**

7. An ADHD evaluation should take approximately:

a. fifteen minutes if the child is hyperactive

b. one hour under most circumstances

c. **three to four hours**

d. ten hours or more

8. In a doctor's office, the child with ADHD will usually:

a. show his ADHD symptoms quickly

b. **sit still**

c. not leave his mother's side

d. tear the place apart

9. Children with ADHD usually respond better to their:

a. **fathers than to their mothers**

b. mothers than to their fathers

c. babysitters than to their teachers

d. none of the above

10. Research has shown that ADHD is primarily:

a. learned or acquired as the child grows up

b. **hereditary**

c. caused by ineffective parenting

d. caused by diet

11. If a child has a sibling who has ADHD, that child's chances of also having ADHD are:

a. zero

b. 100 percent

c. 70 percent

d. **30 percent**

12. Which is *not* a useful prognostic indicator with ADHD?
    a. socioeconomic status
    b. hobbies
    c. intelligence
    d. social skills

There is no correct answer here! These are all useful prognostic indicators.

13. Which is a possible cause of ADHD in some kids?
    a. poor sleep
    b. sugar
    c. allergies
    d. **lead**

14. Kids with ADHD can often sit and concentrate in situations that are:
    a. **novel**
    b. **interesting**
    c. **intimidating**
    d. **one-on-one**

15. Impulsivity refers to:
    a. thinking without acting
    b. acting and carefully thinking
    c. postponing action
    d. **acting without thinking**

16. With peers, kids with ADHD often tend to be:
    a. indifferent
    b. **intrusive**
    c. too placid
    d. too cooperative

17. Externalizing disorders:
    a. don't bother anyone
    b. bother oneself but not others
    c. **bother others but not oneself**
    d. bother only parents

18. Another way of looking at ADHD is to see it as:
    a. a problem with self-abuse
    b. **a problem with self-control**
    c. a problem with thinking straight
    d. a problem with depression

19. What percentage of kids with ADHD will sit still in a doctor's office?
    a. 10 percent
    b. 40 percent
    c. **80 percent**
    d. 95 percent

20. A developmental history is critical to diagnosis and should be carefully taken from:
    a. **the child**
    b. **the teacher**
    c. close relatives from outside the family
    d. **the parents**

So what's your ADHD IQ? Our suggestion is this: if you have a child with ADHD, you should aspire to score 85 percent or better (seventeen to twenty items correct) on the test. Consider sharing this test with other family members, friends, or your child's teacher.

Counseling

The issue of counseling for ADHD has many sides to it. Who is going to be counseled, children and/or parents? Are children with ADHD good counseling or psychotherapy candidates? What about counseling for comorbid conditions, such as anxiety or conduct disorder? How do education about ADHD and counseling work together?

Counseling for Children with ADHD

There is some controversy about counseling kids with ADHD. Many people feel that these children are very much in need of counseling or psychotherapy. After all, these children can be problems to themselves and others, and the prognosis for untreated ADHD is guarded.

Just because a strategy looks like it's needed and appears logical, however, doesn't always make it a good idea. Two factors make counseling children with ADHD difficult. First of all, the very characteristics that characterize ADHD can also make these kids poor candidates for counseling. Are you a good counseling candidate, for example, if you don't want to see the therapist, blame everyone else for your problems, don't pay attention well during a session, and, finally, forget everything that was discussed after you get home? Probably not.

Second, research has shown that the core symptoms of ADHD—impaired concentration, impulsivity, and hyperactivity—simply do not respond to counseling or psychotherapy.[1] You just can't make these things change through talking therapies. Many parents have learned this lesson the hard way: "He's seen Dr. Matthews every week for the last two years, but he's just as disorganized and restless as he was to begin with!" It's very hard to say something verbally to a child with ADHD in a doctor's office that is going to change his behavior during the other 167 hours in the week.

Yet it is essential for kids with ADHD (and their parents) to see some professionals periodically as they are growing up. The visits certainly do not need to be weekly, and what is actually done during the visits may not really qualify as counseling or psychotherapy in the strict sense. The counselor is really more of a monitor or treatment supervisor, and he or she may serve several functions. These include moral support, continuing education about ADHD, mediation, problem prevention, and the fine tuning of the overall treatment plan.

In a world that seems to be continually critical of his every action, a child with ADHD having someone who listens sympathetically and points out his good qualities can be like a breath of fresh air. A good relationship with the doctor also helps the child cooperate with the treatment. The therapist can help educate the child about attention deficit as much as is possible. In fact, it is often better if this information comes from an outsider rather than from one of the child's parents. From time to time, the counselor may also help mediate disputes between the child and his parents, which can cover issues such as homework (at age ten), the use of the car (at age sixteen), or chores (at any age).

How can you determine the extent to which a child can benefit from this kind of supervision/monitoring/counseling process? Several factors can give you a rough idea. First of all, the age of the child is important. The cognitive and language skills of a twelve-year-old, for example, make them more likely to benefit than a six-year-old. Second, how well does the child relate to or get along with this particular professional? Some kids are defensive because they see the office visits as simply another embarrassing admission that they have a problem. Other children see the therapist as the only person who ever treats them nicely.

An important consideration that can affect decisions about counseling for a child with ADHD is the extent to which comorbid conditions are present. We mentioned before that prevention—or at least management—of comorbid conditions was one of our treatment goals. Some comorbid conditions can improve the likelihood of counseling being useful, while others reduce this potential for benefit.

> ## Key Concept
> An important consideration that can affect decisions about counseling for a child with ADHD is the extent to which comorbid conditions are present.

Comorbid *DSM-5* disorders that may actually improve therapy prospects for kids with ADHD include depression and the anxiety disorders. We know that these conditions can respond quite favorably to talk therapies (as well as certain medications). On the other hand, the disorders that make for poorer therapeutic prospects include oppositional defiant and conduct disorders. Even though kids with ODD and CD still need therapeutic monitoring and supervision, these children are very tough to talk with profitably.

Counseling for Parents

When it comes to parents of kids with ADHD, providing good information about ADHD has to be done. But educating parents about ADHD can evoke a good deal of emotion in the recipients of this new knowledge. Reliable information about ADHD will affect people's thoughts not only about the disorder but also about themselves, as well as the whole treatment procedure. Learning the facts about ADHD, therefore, is going to be intimately involved with—and sometimes indistinguishable from—psychotherapy or counseling, especially for parents.

A good example of this information/therapy mixture is what we sometimes call the no-fault idea about ADHD. When a professional explains that ADHD has a hereditary base to it that no one in the family—child or parent—could have changed, this person is essentially saying that ADHD is no one's fault. The no-fault idea has two major implications. The first is that parents no longer need to crucify themselves with guilt about what they think they did to produce this troublesome behavior in their offspring. The guilt that parents have been feeling, however, is tenacious, and it has been long standing. Guilt doesn't just suddenly evaporate, so the job of counseling is to learn, practice, and reinforce correct ways of thinking until these new ideas become habitual.

The second implication about attributions of fault is that the ADHD isn't the child's fault either. Children with ADHD did not grow up with the goal of torturing their parents and making them miserable. Here, the no-fault idea can reduce the amount of anger parents feel toward their children, but it won't get rid of all the anger. Parents will still get annoyed with their child's behavior.

Parents must also understand that the no-fault idea is not to be used as an excuse by any child for his behavior. Suppose one day, a young child with ADHD is sitting on top of—and pounding on—his little sister. His parents confront him. He responds by saying, "I can't help it, 'cause I have ADHD. I have a problem with emotional overarousal, impulsivity, and low frustration tolerance!" This self-serving proclamation is just an excuse, and discipline should follow. Counseling, emotional adjustments, and behavior management are all intertwined.

Another example of education and counseling working together has to do with parents' perceptions of their children and self-esteem. During a session with parents, for example, a therapist may say, "Your son who does not have ADHD is getting straight As. Your daughter who has ADHD is getting straight Ds. In your opinion, which child is working harder?"

The parents are told that, yes, their son without ADHD is working hard and is a wonderful child. But their daughter has to get up every morning and go to school—an activity she despises. It is actually much harder for her than for their son. What is required from her every day is a kind of courage that her brother has never had to experience. Parents are taught to look at the world through the eyes of their child diagnosed with ADHD, rather than seeing reality only from the perspective of frustrated parental expectations.

This same idea can be communicated to a boy or girl with ADHD. The message may go something like this: "Look, I'm not here to feel sorry for you. You have ADHD, and it's your job to handle it as well as you can. But I'll tell you one thing. I'll give you credit for guts. I know how much you dislike school, but you still go every day and do most of what you're supposed to. It takes a lot of effort to do something you hate all the time."

After parents are taught to begin to see their child a little differently, they need to learn to apply this same reasoning to themselves. They didn't ask to have a child with ADHD, and they certainly didn't ask for all the extra work, aggravation, and heartbreak that often goes along with that diagnosis. Yet they too continue to do what must be done from day to day, just helping to keep the kid afloat. This includes the mundane parental operations of driving, cooking, laundry, and purchasing necessities like toothpaste and clothes.

The job also includes the harder tasks that go along with having a child with special needs, such as going to meetings with teachers and staff, seeing counselors, and perhaps putting up with large doses of embarrassment at family picnics. No one will give any parent a medal for doing these things, but perhaps they should.

The stress of raising and living with a child with ADHD takes a lot out of a parent. As mentioned before, parents of children with ADHD, as a group, show a higher incidence of problems such as depression, alcoholism, antisocial personality, anxiety disorders, and adult ADHD. Parents also get involved in more marital discord, as well as separation and divorce.

These problems are not all caused, of course, by the existence of the child's challenges. But when parents do have one of the problems just mentioned, counseling and medication are often indicated. Often, marital counseling for both parents together can help a lot. This is another example of the importance of regular visits to mental health counselors. Treatment can help immensely with a parent's individual adjustment, help stabilize the marriage and the family, and provide more support and structure for the child with ADHD.

One of the biggest oversights in treating these kids is not treating the psychological problems of the parents. Too many therapists tiptoe around a parent's depression or drinking, for example, with the result that the effectiveness of treatment is reduced considerably.

As you know from looking at the previous outline of treatment, there's more to dealing with ADHD than education, counseling, and the supervision/monitoring of therapy. Medication is usually very helpful, but so is training, for both parents and kids. In the next two chapters, we'll look at the issue of training parents in the behavior management of children with ADHD. Then we'll examine the challenging job of training these kids in self-control and social skills.

9
SELF-CONTROL AND SOCIAL SKILLS TRAINING

AS WAS DISCUSSED IN the previous chapter, counseling children with ADHD is sometimes difficult, but it is not impossible. Regular follow-up over the years is essential to good treatment and good outcomes. I often view the counseling process less as psychotherapy and more as education, moral support, mediation, and monitoring.

Outside of office visits, however, parents often wonder if there are activities or therapies that might help to reduce ADHD symptoms. Is there any way to cure ADHD? In this chapter, we'll examine efforts to help children with ADHD improve their self-control. We'll also explore social skills training programs designed to teach kids with ADHD to get along better with peers. In chapter 10, we'll look at complementary and alternative medicine (CAM) approaches to ADHD. Then in chapter 12, we'll conclude by describing exactly what all this teaches us about the treatment of this disorder.

Self-Control Training
Is it possible to train kids with ADHD to reduce their symptoms of

hyperactivity, inattentiveness, and impulsivity in a way that improves their self-control? How would training be different from counseling or supervision? Training would be more than just talking. It would involve putting children through repeated exercises of different kinds that would help them learn new skills. Training might be a bit like learning to play the piano, and it would mean lots of practice. But perhaps practice and repetition might be what it takes to get the idea through to these kids.

Not so many years ago, there was a good deal of excitement and optimism about self-control training for impulsive youngsters with ADHD. Some of this self-control training fell under the category of cognitive behavior therapy (CBT). The cognitive part of CBT referred to the hope that children with ADHD could be taught to think differently before acting. The behavioral part of CBT referred to the hope that these children could be taught to act differently—at least in part because of their new thoughts.[1]

CBT techniques often involved what was called self-instruction training or self-guided talk. This approach took the point of view that the child's difficulties with self-control resulted from a lack of an internal language. A child without ADHD, for example, might be more naturally skilled at talking to herself, be better able to anticipate the consequences of her actions, and then be able to make a good decision about what to do or not do. "If I hit her, I'll get in trouble." Some CBT techniques, therefore, tried to teach the child diagnosed with ADHD how to create and use this internal dialogue.

Although all this sounded logical, the results of training in self-guided talk were disappointing. One of the primary problems was that children with ADHD "forgot to remember" to use the strategy. Even though children were able to repeat the process back to their trainer, when the time actually came to use the tactic, the new strategy was the furthest thing from their mind. This type of forgetfulness is common in kids with ADHD.

Interest in CBT or self-talk approaches was followed by interest in other kinds of self-control or self-regulation training. One type of training included self-monitoring and related self-reinforcement approaches.[2]

Unfortunately, these self-regulation strategies also ran into significant problems.[3] Although positive effects often occurred in the treatment settings, these effects did not generalize to classrooms different from the one in which the tactics were first learned. Some type of adult environmental management still seemed to be necessary. In other words, adults had to help kids with generalization, or the new training would not take effect.

More recently, attempts at self-control training have taken a somewhat different form. By redefining the problem as one of executive functioning, some programs have tried to train kids to improve their functioning in areas such as working memory. The results? The now familiar but frustrating pattern: some change is seen in treatment settings, but there is little or no generalization of new skills elsewhere.[4]

Social Skills Training

One of the most heartbreaking experiences for parents of children with ADHD is to see their child rejected by his or her peers. The ability to get along with others is not only an enjoyable part of life, but it also helps determine how successful a person will be in most endeavors, such as school, career, and family. Consequently, the level of social skills is one of the most important prognostic indicators for what a child's life will be like once they're adults.

When it was first attempted, social skills training employed systematic approaches, which provided for the introduction and mastery of individual skills in a supportive environment. The goal was the generalization of these skills to other settings. For some time, it was believed that the most straightforward treatment was to tell the child what to do in situations identified as problematic; show him or her how to do it; and have the child practice the skill before using the strategies in real life. Parents and teachers could then take advantage of opportunities to strengthen the new behavior. Some social skills training groups lasted from about eight to fifteen weeks.[5]

In social skills training groups, positive social behaviors were first identified, like introducing yourself, sharing, and compromising.

Then these different behaviors were discussed. Each skill might be dealt with separately. Finally, the children were involved in role-play situations, where they acted out examples of good compromising and bad compromising.[6]

Children were reinforced regularly for their cooperation; during the group sessions, there were frequent breaks. Because the transfer of new skills to the nongroup real world was a concern, homework assignments were given to the children for further practice. Sometimes, parents and teachers were also informed of the skills kids were learning, and suggestions were given to the adults for reinforcing these behaviors when they occurred.

Once again, however, the results of social skills training were disappointing.[7] Ironically, in the groups themselves, kids with ADHD were pretty good when it came to defining skills, describing bad behavior, generating new behavioral alternatives, and role-playing. As it was with the CBT techniques, however, in their everyday lives, these children just didn't seem to remember to use the new thoughts and skills that had been discussed and suggested to them—even if it was still the same day! As we have just seen with self-control training, logic and necessity do not by themselves make treatments work.

What's the Problem Here?

Let's reflect on the frustrations with self-control and social skills training for kids with ADHD, see what we can conclude, and then see what we can do.

> **Key Concept**
> Children with ADHD do not seem to generalize learning from a training situation to other real-life situations.

First of all, children with ADHD do not seem to generalize learning from a training situation to other real-life situations. It's important to keep in mind, however, that they *do improve* in the training condition.

Second, many experts feel that efforts such as social skills training are not effective because they are not defining the problem correctly to start with. These people believe that the problem with kids who have ADHD represents a *performance* deficit rather than a *knowledge* deficit. In other words, children with ADHD know what they should do (the knowledge is there), but when the time comes to do it, they don't do it (the performance is not there).

Why not? Because the basic symptoms of ADHD—inattentiveness, hyperactivity, and impulsivity—take over in the heat of the current moment. Ask one of these children, after an unfortunate social encounter, what he should have done, and he may correctly tell you, "I shouldn't have interrupted and been so loud." Although he is correct, this knowledge does him little good. He "forgot" to stop, look, and listen, and then respond.

Then why do these kids with ADHD do better in the actual training situations? Because both behavior management and medication (more about these later), which research shows can help a lot with self-control and social functioning, are being used in the situations where improvements in ADHD-like behavior are desired. Some experts refer to this as the *point of performance*.[8]

Although it usually doesn't totally normalize the social behavior of kids with ADHD, medication can help to reduce their intrusive and irritating actions and to increase their ability to listen and think *before* acting. And when a behavior management program is in place, and a child with ADHD knows exactly how and when the adults in a situation are going to respond to his behavior, he will often do better. But the adults have to be there!

Third, a final problem affecting social skills in particular has to do with the notion of a child's reputation. It's a sad fact that once a bad reputation has been established, it is awfully hard to get rid of. Also making matters worse is the well-established truth that even when a person improves their behavior, their bad reputation tends to remain in place.

Other Alternatives for Social Skills Training

Even though the jury is still out, many creative and compassionate minds continue to work on the problem of social skills training. When it comes to these issues, both parents and professionals feel they have no choice but to try to do something. If you look at the problem from the perspective of treating the school or treating the classroom rather than the child, there may be more room for optimism.

School-Based Programs

A child with ADHD engages in irritating and aggressive behavior, thus creating a bad reputation within their peer group. You might also consider training the child's peers to be more welcoming and accepting and setting up school-wide social skills programs. Work is being undertaken, for example, to set up school-wide social skills programs where all children are exposed to a basic philosophy of interpersonal relations as well as to specific classroom interventions.[9]

All teachers, for example, might be required to participate in a school program that does not allow rejection of others or bullying. That might mean teachers need to work on not modeling rejecting behaviors toward a difficult child they do not like. Kids quickly pick up on adult attitudes and can use them as permission for their own hostile actions.

Problem solving and conflict resolution exercises might also be incorporated into the classroom in some schools. One advantage of this is that children with ADHD are not singled out as needing special help. All kids are exposed to the activities. A disadvantage may be that other children benefit more from the exercises than kids with an ADHD diagnosis do, and other kids may not need the practice as much in the first place.

Parents as Models and Trainers

Some individuals have pointed out that the apparent failings of self-control and social skills training efforts with children who have ADHD need to be put in a different perspective. These people ask if it is really fair to expect major behavioral changes in this difficult bunch of kids in such a short a period of time (e.g., fifteen weeks).

Perhaps not. On the other hand, we do know that ADHD symptoms tend to moderate with age. Children with ADHD tend to become somewhat less hyperactive and impulsive, although they may remain just as inattentive and disorganized. In a sense, then, they do mature, even though this maturing process can progress much more slowly than it does in neurotypical children. So can social skills training help to foster and improve, perhaps speed up just a little, this maturation over the long haul?

Possibly, but it won't happen in one self-control or social skills training group or one summer camp experience. These activities may provide some useful booster sessions every now and then, but the real, everyday trainers are going to be parents. For one thing, kids learn a lot through modeling, and they are definitely going to imitate the behavior of their parents. If parents exercise reasonable self-control, then their children will *tend* to do the same. If parents model good social skills, then their kids will *tend* to do the same.

This is another reason why it is important to treat parents as well as the child with ADHD. Parents themselves often suffer the effects of ADHD and disorders such as anxiety and depression. These problems can interfere with their effectively modeling good self-control and effective social interactions.

In addition to being *models* for their kids, parents must also be *trainers*. You really don't have much choice. Time with parents offers ample opportunities for training. Training means not only discipline and modeling, but also finding friendly ways to prompt and reinforce your child's efforts at self-regulation and positive social interaction.

Here's an example. We know that kids with ADHD run into more social problems in unstructured situations. Research also tells us that children with ADHD, especially ADHD-C, often do much better in social interactions with the help of medication.[10] So parents might think of themselves as permanent social engineers.

What some parents do is set up a get-together with another child— often someone from their class or neighborhood. But the other child doesn't just come over to play with the two children doing whatever they want. Instead, the child with ADHD takes his medication sometime before the potential friend shows up. Then playtime is structured. Perhaps the two kids watch a DVD or go out with a parent for ice cream or to a ballgame. The visit is short, and activities like competitive games are avoided. Parents may have to experiment to try to find the structure or activity that makes the experience pleasant for both children. Parents also acknowledge and reinforce appropriate self-control and positive social behaviors when their child shows them. This might involve charting, positive reinforcers, and a short, pleasant post-play debriefing session between parent and child.

Could you set up something like this once a week for your child? It's a fair amount of work, but if you did it once a week, in one year, your child would have had perhaps fifty positive social experiences. The other possibility is he might make a friend. My opinion is that just having one friend by itself might do more good for the skills and self-esteem of a child diagnosed with ADHD than a hundred counseling sessions or training groups.

Medication and Social Skills

Some pediatricians tell parents that stimulant medication for ADHD should only be used for school. This attitude is unfortunate, and it is one that does a great disservice to many kids with ADHD. Today, research has made it perfectly clear that medications help most children with ADHD in social situations—especially children with ADHD-C.[11] Some people say, "That's ridiculous. How can a pill teach a skill?" This comment misses the point. Remember that with ADHD, the problem is not knowledge but performance. Medication can help these children stop, look, and listen and then perform properly using the knowledge they already have. The pill does not teach the skill; the pill helps the child access the skill.

I have two final comments about medication. ADHD is a challenge 365 days a year. It does not go away on weekends or during the summer. Most kids do better when they use medication during these times also, rather than just when school is in session. Also, I mentioned before that early detection (diagnosis) is a positive predictive indicator. I also mentioned that bad reputations are hard to shake. Imagine a little girl with ADHD-C who is diagnosed at age five and starts taking medication before her first day in kindergarten. If she responds very well socially to the meds, then she has a good chance of getting off to a good start in school and not having a bad reputation with her peers by the time she hits second or third grade.

10

CHALLENGES WITH ALTERNATIVE THERAPIES FOR ADHD

YEARS AGO, WHEN WE (parents and therapists) were all working hard to get our national support groups, Children and Adults with Attention Deficit Disorder (CHADD) and the Attention Deficit Disorder Association (ADDA), going, those of us with children diagnosed with ADHD dreamed of a day when useful and accurate knowledge about ADHD would be spread throughout the country. We hoped that, at a future date, children and adults with ADHD would be diagnosed efficiently, and good treatment would be available.

In a sense, that day has already come. But what came along with it—which we did not expect—was a national prejudice against the diagnosis of ADHD and an even stronger prejudice against medication treatment for this disorder. This prejudice isn't as bad as it used to be, but it still interferes with the application of useful and well-founded information about the problem of ADHD.

The prejudice against diagnosis was at least partially based on the fact that ADHD usually involves irritating behavior, and placing a diagnosis on that felt to some like we were "making excuses" for obnoxious people who simply had little willpower. The medication prejudice was due in part to reservations about giving drugs to kids and in part to the seemingly illogical paradox of using stimulants to reduce hyperactivity.

Since ADHD is so prevalent, and there has always been much opposition to medication treatment, there has been an explosion of alternative treatments, or what some people call complementary and alternative medicine (CAM). It has been estimated that over half of the parents of children with ADHD use one or more CAM treatments, which they do not usually reveal to their pediatricians.[1]

High Stakes and Confusion about What Works

One of the problems with the fields of physical and mental health is the challenge of trying to determine what kinds of treatments work with what particular problems. Unfortunately, you often hear of many different kinds of treatments that—according to some people—work for many different kinds of problems. In the areas of psychology and psychiatry especially, there are many more claims of effectiveness made than there are legitimate approaches.

This proliferation of claims is partly due to the fact that placebo effects are more rampant in mental health than in physical medicine. Placebo effects occur when someone apparently "gets better" because he thinks (or his parents think) he is being treated with an effective procedure. Placebo effects usually don't last very long, and with ADHD, these effects occur less often than they do with other psychological problems. One research study, for example, on placebo effects with depression concluded that placebos could reproduce about 75 percent of the improvement from an antidepressant drug.[2] With ADHD, however, these artificial effects usually don't exceed 10 percent.[3]

Adults who are constantly frustrated by kids with ADHD—and who are nervous about medication—often are anxious to climb on a new treatment bandwagon. And for a while, these adults may see a new treatment as being helpful when in fact it isn't really changing anything. Parents who are willing to go to the trouble of trying some new kind of diet, for example, may also inadvertently do other things (such as use more positive reinforcement) that may help their child do better for a while. Or, because of all the effort they have put in, parents may perceive their child as doing better when in fact his behavior may not be much different.

Sorting It All Out

How can you tell if an alternative treatment for ADHD is likely to be a waste of time? Generally, unless you're willing to read all the literature and go to all the conferences on the subject, it can be quite difficult. You almost always have to rely on someone else's opinion. If you're a parent, you pretty much have to rely on the professionals, and even if you're a professional, you still have to rely on other professionals.

Fortunately, professionals write a lot and even argue in their writings and research. What is good about all this squabbling is that if somebody comes up with a new treatment idea, they had better be able to prove that it works, and the new idea had better be able to stand the test of time. Other professionals—even those who didn't develop the idea—must also do studies that show the treatment works.

Good research is careful and painstaking. It requires careful selection of subjects, a double-blind setup where people don't know what's real treatment and what's placebo, the existence of a control group (those who get a placebo), and replication in which other investigators have to get the same results.

All this research and arguing back and forth is published in professional journals. All this disagreement may sound tedious and petty, but it serves a purpose. After a while, it's possible to get a sense of the state of the art and to learn what works and what doesn't. According to scientific literature that involves carefully designed and controlled studies, the strategies that stand the test of time will be recommended. Other approaches will fall by the wayside or will eventually fall into the category of what I call controversial and idiosyncratic therapies.

How do you know if a proposed treatment falls into this controversial category? It's not always easy, but there are several ways. One is that the theoretical basis of the method doesn't fit with modern scientific knowledge. Another way to tell is if there are claims that the technique is effective for a broad range of rather poorly defined problems. In addition, adverse effects of the new method are often minimized, since the therapy may emphasize natural methods such as diet, vitamins, or bodily manipulations. Finally, the publication of the therapy may appear in the popular media sources rather than in scientific journals. Later, controlled scientific studies that don't support the method will be discounted due to so-called bias or the alleged unwillingness of the scientific community to accept new ideas.

Alternative Therapies

While there are numerous alternative techniques, there are several that fall under the category of controversial and unproven: megavitamins, chiropractic treatment, sensory integration training, yoga, meditation, acupuncture, homeopathy, and massage. These treatments have only spotty anecdotal information (e.g., "it seemed to work for my roommate's cousin") and few or no well-designed, placebo-controlled studies indicating that the treatment did some good.[4] Useful treatments, on the other hand, have many controlled studies that have been replicated by other controlled studies, and numerous positive anecdotes back them up.

There are some alternative techniques that show promise but don't yet have substantial research to back them up.

Biofeedback

Biofeedback uses certain instruments to provide feedback to individuals regarding their current physiological states. People can learn, for example, to alter brain waves, muscle tone, and heart rate in ways that can help produce greater relaxation and other healthier modes of functioning. It's the brain wave alteration possibilities that got some people thinking about ADHD. Proponents of biofeedback have been claiming positive effects on ADHD symptoms (not just behavior management) for quite a while, but they can't seem to produce good controlled studies and then replicate them.

Caffeine and Nicotine

Caffeine and nicotine are both central nervous system (CNS) stimulants that have the potential to act like methylphenidate (generic form of Ritalin) or amphetamine when it comes to ADHD. Those of us clinicians who have worked with ADHD for many years have heard a lot of stories about the benefits on concentration of these easy-to-get substances. Stories about Uncle Jim who got himself through college on coffee and cigarettes before he was diagnosed with ADHD are very common.

Research on caffeine has shown positive effects in helping with ADHD symptoms, but the effects tend to be somewhat erratic and short-lived.[5] This is not surprising, since the administration and dosing of the drug is hard to measure. Nicotinic agents have also shown some promise in some studies, but these have not as yet been replicated, and so the therapies have not been used.[6] Interest remains, however, in the possibilities of gums, patches, or even electronic cigarettes.

Dietary Changes

As was mentioned earlier, it is possible that a small number of children with ADHD are diet sensitive in such a way that certain foods or additives either make them feel bad or help worsen their behavior. These substances don't cause ADHD, but they may aggravate behavior.[7] Elimination diets often focus on the elimination of dairy, gluten, citrus fruits, corn products, processed foods, and sometimes artificial food colors from the diet.

Elimination diets are a lot of work and need to be done carefully. A good medical evaluation should be done beforehand. Parents have to decide how much control they can have over a child's diet and also what the rest of the family is going to be eating while the child is on the diet. It's best to eliminate one thing at a time, and results can take several months to appear—if they are going to appear at all. The whole process should be supervised by a competent dietician.

In cases where medication for ADHD is already being used, has been carefully titrated, and children and their families are not seeing positive benefits, then an elimination diet may be considered. If an elimination diet is followed *instead* of medication treatment, keep in mind that it may take a while, and the chances of success are not certain. The dietary trial, therefore, is delaying the use of a powerful, evidence-based treatment.

Omega-3 Fatty Acids

Several well-controlled studies have found small but significant benefits for children diagnosed with ADHD from dietary supplementation using polyunsaturated fatty acids (PUFAs).[8] Using omega-3 fatty acid supplements, positive treatment effects were found regarding both inattentive and hyperactive symptoms. For children who were already taking stimulant medication, PUFA supplementation did not add much extra in terms of symptom reduction. The thinking at present, therefore, is that PUFAs may be more useful when medication treatment is not providing good results.[9]

Timid Professionals

Perhaps because of the national prejudice against ADHD, in my opinion, mental health professionals, educators, and physicians have become too timid about making the diagnosis of ADHD, recommending legitimate therapies, and discouraging the use of unproven therapies. A doctor might say, for example, "My diagnosis of your seven-year-old is ADHD, combined type. I understand you want to try megavitamins for a while. That's your decision, and that's fine. Let me know how it goes."

No, it's not fine. Parents have two critical—but limited—resources. One of these resources is money. Diagnosing, tutoring, counseling, books about ADHD, and medication can be expensive. Most families don't have a lot of money to throw around.

A second important, limited resource is time. The outcomes for untreated ADHD are scary. Mental health professionals and parents must do the best they can as soon as they can for kids by using what has been proven to work. Otherwise, a valuable period of a child's growing-up time may be robbed of its full potential, and untreated ADHD will do further damage.

I saw a family many years ago about their third-grade son. His grades were bad, he had no friends, and he was very difficult to manage at home. I diagnosed ADHD and recommended medication, among other things. The family politely declined the medication. I explored their feelings about this treatment, but they did not change their mind.

The family returned three years later. Their son was in sixth grade. The situation was about the same: his grades were still bad, he had no friends, and things were awful at home. By then, the parents were willing to try medication. The boy responded very well to the medication. After taking it regularly for a while, his grades jumped, and he became easier to get along with.

The parents' first reaction to this wonderful outcome? They cried. Why? Because their boy had lost three years of his growing-up time. Those three years had been bad, and they were irretrievable.

So What Does Work?

Over the years, controlled research has repeatedly confirmed the value of three kinds of interventions for children with ADHD: behavior management training for parents, medication for the child with ADHD, and specific classroom interventions to help the child with ADHD in school.[10] In the next chapters, we'll examine these approaches. These strategies work, but it's important to remember what "work" means. Work does not mean cure. Instead, works means that while these treatments are in place, ADHD symptoms and impairment are suppressed (often a lot), so that kids, parents, and teachers have enjoyable, successful days. Those positive experiences are then stored permanently in the memory banks of all people involved.

11

BEHAVIOR MANAGEMENT AT HOME AND IN PUBLIC

IMAGINE YOU'VE HAD YOUR child sent through a thorough diagnostic evaluation, and it has been determined that your son or daughter has ADHD. You've started the process of educating yourself about this disorder, and you have chosen a therapist to help you with the treatment process. Your therapist very likely will be a licensed counselor, clinical social worker, or psychologist who is trained in the diagnosis and treatment of ADHD. There are a lot of good pediatricians and child psychiatrists, but these doctors usually don't have the time to act as the coleader with you as part of your child's ADHD treatment team.

In this chapter, we'll discuss behavior management for ADHD at home and also in public. While we don't have room in one chapter to describe all the details involved in ADHD behavior management, we will try to provide some guidelines about what needs to be included in such a program. These guidelines will give you an idea of what changes you'll need to make, and they'll also help you select a discipline method, allowing you to guide your child toward appropriate behavior in a variety of circumstances.

When looking at discipline programs for ADHD, remember that you should have goals for the present and the future. For the present, you want to enjoy your son or daughter, you want to prevent the ADHD comorbidities (such as ODD, CD, drug abuse, anxiety, and depression), and you want to enjoy—separate from your child diagnosed with ADHD—yourself and the rest of your family. For the future, you want your child to grow up and successfully leave home.

The good news is that the solid efforts you put into behavior management will simultaneously help accomplish *all* those goals. The bad news is that managing the behavior of kids with ADHD can be very challenging. It will not always go perfectly, but your friendly mental health professional should provide the expertise, supervision, and moral support you need to get through even the most difficult times.

The Challenges

There are three unique challenges that make disciplining kids with ADHD especially demanding: the 30 percent rule, countertransference, and the point of performance problem.

The 30 percent rule states that from an emotional and behavioral maturity point of view, kids with ADHD will usually be about 30 percent behind their peers.[1] A six-year-old with ADHD, for example, will behave more like a neurotypical four-year-old, a twelve-year-old with ADHD like a neurotypical eight-year-old, and so on. One of the lessons for parents based on the 30 percent rule is that you can't expect normal behavior from a child with ADHD. You want to set your expectations realistically. Your child will keep progressing and maturing, but there will always be this maturity gap.

> **Key Concept**
>
> There are three unique challenges that make disciplining kids with ADHD especially demanding: the 30 percent rule, countertransference, and the point of performance problem.

The second challenge for behavior management of kids with ADHD is what we call countertransference. This is a concept borrowed from psychotherapy. Countertransference refers to a psychotherapist's feelings toward their own client and their client's behavior.[2] If a patient makes a therapist feel overly sympathetic or overly angry, for example, those feelings can interfere with good treatment. Therapists are not machines; they are people too.

When children have ADHD, a big problem is that their externalizing behaviors are often irritating to others. This, as mentioned before, is one of the causes for the national prejudice against ADHD. It is difficult to feel sympathetic toward a person of any age who annoys you consistently. If, on the other hand, you have a nine-year-old daughter who is depressed and sad because you just got divorced, your heart is likely to go out to her, and you want to help. The misbehaviors in children with ADHD often create aggravation in parents and other authority figures. Unfortunately, aggravation can inspire a desire to punish more than a desire to help. Consistent irritation makes good discipline harder for parents and teachers to implement. So to be a good disciplinarian, in other words, you need to be aware of your own feelings and how they affect your behavior.

The final behavior management challenge is the point of performance problem. Because of the ever-present symptoms of inattention, impulsivity, and hyperactivity, it's very hard to teach a child with ADHD a behavior or skill and then expect them to remember it on their own and to apply it in a new situation. The therapies that work best—parent training, classroom management, and medication—provide direction and assistance to kids *at the time and place in which the child has to perform.* It's true that children with ADHD will gradually expand their abilities to function independently as they get older, but the point of performance law has to be taken into account when planning any interventions for them.

Defining a Parent's Behavior Management Job

Research shows that parent training works—it makes for better child behavior and less stress at home.[3] In my experience, parents who successfully go through parent training feel much better about themselves as parents, and their relationships with their spouses or partners improve.

In this section, we'll discuss a way of organizing the job of parenting a child diagnosed with ADHD. Then I'll give you some ideas about the kinds of strategies you'll need to learn to carry out that job. When you have a child with ADHD, you will have to put in quite a bit of physical, emotional, and attitudinal effort, but you will find it's worth it.

Let's take a look at how one might define the parenting job in general. Here's a list of some of the problems/issues that have to be managed with all kids in a typical day or week:

- arguing
- up and out in the morning
- whining
- going to bed
- yelling

- eating
- sibling rivalry
- homework
- tantrums
- picking up
- disrespect

- chores
- pouting
- cleaning room
- lying

That's already a lot—and it's not even everything! Add ADHD to the mix, and you've got quite a challenge for yourself. Whether you're the parent of a child with ADHD or a parent of neurotypical kids, it's very important that *you have a strategy for each and every one of those problems.* For your strategy to be effective in the long run, it can't involve unproductive tactics like arguing, yelling, and nagging, which are expressions of the countertransference/anger problem just discussed.

Let's look at the list of issues again, but reorganize it, so that every item is in one of two categories: (1) unpleasant behavior that you want your kids to stop, and (2) positive behavior you want your kids to start and finish. Here are the two *new* lists:

UNPLEASANT BEHAVIOR (STOP)	POSITIVE BEHAVIOR (START)
arguing	up and out in the morning
whining	going to bed
yelling	eating
sibling rivalry	homework
tantrums	picking up
disrespect	chores
pouting	cleaning room
lying	

Now, we know kids with ADHD have trouble paying attention and sustaining motivation. The behavior on the two lists above is very different in that regard. For obnoxious behavior (left side), like arguing or teasing, a child has to pay attention to your command or request and then stop the behavior. How long does that take? About one second. It's not a big job.

But for the other list (right side), positive behavior, a child has to not only pay attention to your command, but they must also *start and sustain their performance*. Cleaning a room, for example, might take thirty-five minutes. That's much longer than one second!

So it's easy to see that you might need different strategies for the examples on the left vs. the examples on the right. For suppressing unpleasant behavior, we use crisp, clear commands. In my bestselling book focused entirely on managing child behavior, *1–2–3 Magic*, that means counting to three and giving the child the opportunity to stop the behavior. If the child does not comply, there's a consequence.

For encouraging positive behavior, on the other hand, you might need a prompt (to get attention) plus something else to help sustain the behavior. As is explained in *1–2–3 Magic*, to help a child clean her room, you might also use charts to help the child track her own progress plus artificial reinforcers, such as tokens that can be exchanged for pleasant activities or things.

Strategies You'll Need to Learn

In this section, we're going to briefly introduce you to some of the strategies that will help manage your child with ADHD. This section is a kind of heads-up about what's coming, but it also serves as a kind of attitude adjustment. You may find yourself thinking, "Why can't my kid just do what's he's supposed to? Why do I have to learn all this?" The answer is: because your child has ADHD, and in the long run, you and your family will be a lot happier if you put in the time now mastering new skills. You will be discussing this attitude adjustment—in its many different forms—frequently with your therapist!

Praise and Positive Reinforcement

One of the most effective—and surprisingly difficult—strategies is reinforcing the positive behavior of kids with ADHD. Some frustrated parents might say, "What positive behavior?" It is there. Your job as a parent is to identify it and reinforce it. You can reinforce good behavior physically through smiles, pats on the back, hugs, thumbs-up, or with words like "Nice job!" or "Good work."

The hard part here is this: angry people make noise; happy people keep quiet. When we're angry about someone else's behavior, we're likely to say (or yell) something. When we're happy with their behavior, on the other hand, we often think, "That's what he *should* be doing," or "It's about time!" and then we say nothing. The result: people living with us tend to think they're more of a pain in the neck to us than fun to be around.

> ### Key Concept
> Children with ADHD need a lot of positive reinforcement to help them sustain their positive actions.

Children with ADHD need a lot of positive reinforcement to help them sustain their positive actions. You're going to want your ratio of positive to negative feedback (verbal and nonverbal) to them to be about three to one. Now there's a tough but important job for you!

Being Buffaloed vs. Having Constructive Routines

For any problem behavior (homework) or problem time of the day (evening), you will want to have a routine—a well thought-out method for managing that difficulty. The last thing in the world you want is to be buffaloed (confused or stumped) by the issue. If you don't know what to do in the pinch, you are going to resort to talk, chatter, useless reasoning, arguing, yelling, or even physical abuse. As we'll see in a minute, those are all excellent tactics for creating oppositional defiance disorder (ODD), anxiety, and depression in your child and severely damaging their prognosis.

Good Commands

You're going to learn how to give good commands to your kids. This, for example, is a bad command: "Don't you think it's time to start your homework? OK, honey?" This command reeks of ambivalence and fear. Bad commands also involve parental instructions that a parent has no intention of following up on or instructions that are repeated five times.

You'll learn how to give commands or suggestions and then stick around to reinforce and ensure compliance. You'll find out how important it is for parents to back up each other's directives. You'll also come to understand why command plus explanation is often a much *worse* strategy than a simple command by itself.

MBAs: Minor But Aggravating Behavior

MBAs are the minor but aggravating things that kids do that are somewhat irritating but are not really signs of mental disturbance and are not in need of discipline. When you have kids with ADHD, you'll need to make a list of the kinds of things you're going to *ignore* and not discipline, even if they irritate you a bit. Your list might include restlessness at the dinner table, humming, running in the house, lying down on the bench seat at McDonald's, and perhaps even interrupting. Remember that you don't want to provide a reprimand or a command that you don't intend to follow up on.

Time-Outs

You may have heard negative and positive things about the use of time-outs. The American Academy of Pediatrics recommends the use of time-outs as an effective procedure for undesirable behavior.[4] To be done properly, household (or classroom) rules should first be clear; adults' commands should also be clear and presented in a calm, unemotional manner.

The message of the time-out procedure is this: in this house or classroom, when a certain undesirable behavior occurs, it will be followed by a rest period or break time. Break time gives everyone involved a chance to calm down and forget the whole thing. That's it. The message of time-out is not "You're a rotten kid, and you're driving me nuts!"

What to Do in Public

Even parents who have good discipline strategies at home sometimes crumble when confronted with bad behavior in public. Why? The answer is simple: *the threat of public embarrassment*. First, parents need to adjust their attitude and realize that their kids' future welfare is more important than what you think others are going to think of you when you're out of the house.

When children use bad behavior in public situations, kids often sense parents' anxiety and indecisiveness and proceed to use it against them. This can make for some really awful episodes, especially with behavior like tantrums. A lot of young children get away with things in public that would never be allowed in the privacy of their home. There are a number of tactics to use in public, and you'll need to identify through trial and error which ones work best with your children.

Disrespect

This is a very common discipline concern for all parents, and if you ask parents of children with ADHD, they'll tell you it can be a bigger problem for kids with ADHD than with neurotypical youngsters. Disrespect with ADHD in the picture is not only more frequent, it can also be more vehement due to the symptom of emotional overarousal.

Disrespect directed toward parents can certainly be a legitimate focus of discipline. But one caution is in order. All too often, in a difficult situation, the one who is disrespectful *first* is the parent. The adult's words, tone of voice, and nonverbal manner are harsh and demeaning— often because the child with ADHD is doing something out of line for what feels like the nine millionth time. When the child responds with disrespect, however, he gets nailed. This is a form of entrapment.

Consistency and Parental Diagnoses

Parents of kids with ADHD are more likely to suffer from anxiety, depression, alcohol and substance abuse, and ADHD than are parents whose children do not have ADHD.[5] One of the biggest problems with this unfortunate truth is that having these problems often results in parents being inconsistent in their behavior management strategies. Depression, for example, can make some parents more irritable, with the result that they intervene with their kids too often, too aggressively, and in a degrading manner. Other depressed parents, however, become too passive, and they don't intervene as often or as firmly as they should. One of the things your therapist will help you with, especially in the first few months of getting your behavior program running, is how to stay on the wagon.

Avoiding Comorbid Conditions

You hear a lot of people these days complaining that children are running the show, that five-year-olds are in charge of the house, and that parents refuse to check their children's unruly behavior in public. Parents, it is claimed, just don't exercise their authority anymore. Is this really true?

Although a blanket generalization about parental abdication of authority certainly is not valid, there does appear to be a trend in the direction of increased discomfort with the legitimate use of parental power. In their determination to avoid spanking, yelling, and "because I said so" discipline, and in their concern with "modern parenting" and emotional intelligence, lots of adults these days are becoming conflict avoidant and committed to a philosophy of "Let's talk it out till everyone is happy."

The result is this: in discipline situations, parents are talking too much. Another way of saying this is that parents—in the crunch—all too often engage in *prattle*. The dictionary defines prattle as *talking at length in a foolish or inconsequential way*. I have found that prattle is an excellent way of increasing conflict and also increasing chances of your child developing a comorbid disorder.

Let's look at an example of parental prattle. Fifteen minutes before dinner, seven-year-old Caitlin, who has ADHD, asks her mother for a snack. Here's how the conversation goes:

"Can I have just, like, one of those donuts?"

"Not right now."

"Aw, how come? I'm starving."

"We're eating in just fifteen minutes, honey."

"Yeah, but I really want it."

"I just told you you couldn't have it."

"You never give me anything!"

"I never give you anything? Do you have clothes on? Is there a roof over your head? Am I feeding you in two seconds?"

"You let Allison have ice cream a half hour ago!"

"That was an hour ago. Besides, Allison always finishes her dinner."

"I promise I'll finish my dinner."

"Why do you have to give me a hard time about this, Caitlin?"

"This is stupid! I don't want any of your lousy dinner!"

"Watch that mouth, young lady! You'll eat when I tell you to!"

After line four above ("We're eating in just fifteen minutes..."), this conversation is a power struggle, pure and simple. It may look like two people exchanging ideas, but it is really misbehavior (from the child) and prattle (from the parent) *masquerading as dialogue*.

Unfortunately, modern approaches to parenting (talk it all out till everyone's happy) encourage this kind of misbehavior vs. prattle exchange. Why? Because of the objective (or burden!) these approaches place on parents: in a conflict, you must talk it over until both sides are satisfied; ending *any* interaction with ill will or anger is bad. Mom is also simply buffaloed (not allowed!) by her daughter's protests, so the frustrated parent simply defaults to chattering back.

The ODD Problem

If you don't know when to talk, how to talk, when to stop talking, and what to do after you stop talking with your kids with ADHD, my experience has shown your discipline attempts have a very high probability of producing several important—but bad—effects. The last two involve ADHD comorbidities we're trying to avoid. The bad effects include:

1. a decrease in your children's cooperation on the spot.
2. an increase in kids' testing you and continuing to experiment with manipulation.
3. a much higher risk of oppositional defiant disorder in your children.
4. a much higher risk of emotional and physical abuse from you.
5. regular self-esteem drops in your kids and you, with greater future risk for anxiety and depression in everyone.

In the "Can I have a donut?" exchange above, there is a *big* difference between Mom's feeling about the conversation and Caitlin's. Mom hates the dialogue! She is very unpleasantly aggravated.

What about Caitlin? Caitlin is getting a kick out of hassling her mother. You can't give kids with ADHD (or any kids) everything they want, so part of parenting means you have to irritate your children regularly by saying no and setting limits.

But what if you have a child with ADHD? You discipline them, they get irritated, so they try to annoy you right back. If you then prattle in response, they get multiple opportunities to have fun aggravating you. Repeat these crazy dialogues enough over a period of time, and your child with ADHD gets addicted to revenge, just like someone who smokes cigarette after cigarette gets addicted to smoking. The *DSM-5* tells us that kids with ODD are easily annoyed, resentful, argumentative, touchy, defiant, and spiteful. Because of the patterns of behavior you've helped to enforce, you may have now helped add ODD to your child's diagnostic profile.[6] In a few more years, your child takes their ODD out into the community, and you now have a conduct-disordered child with a bad prognosis.

Talking too much in discipline situations is not an effective solution. One of your most important behavior management skills will be knowing how and when to keep quiet.

Some Behavior Management Alternatives

Your therapist may have their own favorite discipline program for ADHD, but here are several other useful possibilities:

1. *Taking Charge of ADHD* by Russell Barkley
2. *1–2–3 Magic: Effective Discipline for Children 2–12* by Thomas W. Phelan
3. Parent to Parent Program from the organization Children and Adults with Attention Deficit Hyperactivity Disorder (CHADD) (www.chadd.org)

12

MEDICATION FOR ADHD

AT THIS POINT, YOU may already have the following three things in place: (1) a reliable diagnosis of ADHD for your child; (2) a therapist who understands ADHD and who will be the team coleader with you for your treatment program; (3) a beginning perspective on what your behavior management program is going to look like. You may not yet have decided about medication treatment or the kinds of changes or adjustments that are going to have to be made at school. We'll deal with these two issues in the next three chapters.

Medication: Yes or No?

Nearly all parents worry about the idea of their children taking medication for ADHD. Can a medication actually change behavior? If a drug does work, how long will it have to be taken? Can a pill help a child get along with peers or improve performance in sports? Do the pills have to be taken every day? What about side effects? Are these medications addictive? Will they suppress appetite or stunt growth? Will my child look dazed or drugged?

In addition, some parents are suspicious about medication treatment. What is the rationale behind giving a stimulant medication to a hyperactive child or to a restless adult with ADHD in the first place? Does it make sense to give a controlled substance to a child for a behavioral or emotional problem? Isn't this actually encouraging the youngster to use drugs and thus increasing the later risk of substance abuse? Won't that simply result in more trouble down the road?

Parental concern about drug treatment is often heightened by myths about medication treatment and treatment of the subject by TV, newspapers, magazines, radio, and the Internet. Medication myths include the notions that the stimulants used for ADHD do no good at all, that they cause terrible and irreversible side effects, that they are addictive, and that they shouldn't be used after midadolescence.

Unfortunately, media discussion about the use of medication for ADHD also frequently increases parental worries. Presentations that may appear compelling, factual, and objective often show little regard for scientific evidence or longstanding practice. Parents see, read, or hear stories that focus on controversy, on the unusual, and on trouble and misfortune. Positive outcomes do not always make for "good" news.

Balanced against parents' worries about medication, however, is the reality of their child with ADHD. Concerns about drug treatment are abstract thoughts, but their child is flesh and blood. It is often all too obvious that ADHD is dramatically interfering with a child's day-to-day functioning, his overall welfare, and his happiness. To decide whether medication is right for a child with ADHD, parents need to start by obtaining accurate, reliable information.

So the dilemma many parents face is this: drug treatment is scary. It is an unknown quantity—they've never tried it before. ADHD is also scary, but it is a known quantity. Parents realize ADHD is already interfering with school performance, home life, and peer relation-ships. It is taking the joy out of their child's growing up.

Controlled Research on Medication for ADHD

Stimulant medications are usually considered the first-line treat-ment choice for ADHD. The two most commonly used stimulant medications for ADHD, methylphenidate and amphetamine, have been on the market for about seventy years.[1] These drugs help to alleviate the symptoms of ADHD without causing significant harmful side effects.

The Food and Drug Administration (FDA), the government agency that approves prescription medications in the United States, is probably the most conservative organization of its kind in the world. The FDA is not perfect, by any means, but it is very cautious. The agency requires careful research by drug manufacturers before a new compound is approved.

Over three hundred double-blind, placebo controlled studies have been done on the efficacy and side effects of stimulants. What has this research told us? Research has shown that stimulant medication is remarkably effective as well as safe.[2] A stimulant medication prescribed for ADHD is quite helpful about 75 percent of the time. The stimulant will usually help reduce impulsivity and hyperactivity, and it will also help improve concentration by increasing attention span.

> **Key Concept**
> Stimulant medications are usually considered the first-line treatment choice for ADHD.

What's more, when starting medication treatment, if you try two different stimulants in sequence (e.g., methylphenidate then amphetamine) to see which works best, the effectiveness statistic for stimulant treatment rises to over 90 percent of the ADHD population.[3]

What about side effects? When side effects do occur, they are usually mild, and many disappear over a short period of time. Side effects will almost always disappear after the medications are stopped, though discontinuation is not necessary in most cases. Side effects may also disappear if a different stimulant medication is tried. Some common side effects of these types of medication include headache, stomachache, appetite reduction, sadness or irritability, and drowsiness or lethargy.[4]

The MTA Study

The grandfather of all ADHD treatment studies was the Multimodal Treatment of ADHD (MTA) investigation conducted by the National Institute of Mental Health (NIMH), whose initial results were published in 1999. Treatment was provided to 579 seven-to-ten-year-old children in grades one to four who had been diagnosed with ADHD-C. The MTA study did not deal with adolescents or adults.

The MTA studied four kinds of treatment for ADHD. After diagnosis, kids and families were randomly assigned to one of these conditions:

1. intensive medication management alone (this included monthly follow-up visits)
2. behavior management alone (parent training, summer camp for the kids, and school consultation)
3. combined medication plus behavior management
4. community control (treatment conducted by professionals in the community and separate from the MTA study)

The MTA treatments were well-controlled, rigorous, and highly energetic. Some have even described these efforts as heroic, meaning they were a lot more intensive than what you're likely to typically run across in your own community. The treatments went on for fourteen months.

How well did these ADHD treatments work? Success was defined as a score on a follow-up rating scale that indicated symptoms were in the *not at all or just a little* category. At the fourteen-month point, the success rate for the combined treatment was 68 percent, for the medication management it was 56 percent, for behavior management alone it was 34 percent, and for the community comparison group it was 25 percent.[5]

There are several conclusions that can be drawn from the MTA. First, all the treatments worked to some extent. Second, the two treatments that provided the best results both involved intensive (monthly) medication management. Third, the two treatments that parents liked the best (according to posttreatment satisfaction surveys) both involved behavior management (combined behavior/medication treatment and behavior management alone treatment).

There's good news and bad news from the MTA investigation. Most experts take the study as confirmation of the need for multimodal or combined behavioral and drug interventions. Not only did medication help, but also important were parent training and regular visits to some kind of doctor or therapist. That's the kind of treatment plan we outlined earlier, and it's what you will need for you and your child.

The bad news, however, takes us back to the old point of performance problem. When the treatments were phased out and the families followed-up with, the benefits tended to disappear. In other words, with kids with ADHD, you get benefits and changes as long as treatments (behavior management and medication) are in place. *The treatments do not cure ADHD.*

Types of ADHD Medications

Although the MTA study used stimulants, other medications have been used to treat ADHD over the years. Some have been FDA-approved for pediatric use and some have not, even though clinicians have found them useful. In this section, we'll take a quick look at the drugs that have been used to treat ADHD. You'll want your treatment team coleader (even though they may not be a doctor) and your prescribing doctor (pediatrician, child psychiatrist, or neurologist) to be familiar with these medication possibilities. Sometimes, identifying a useful medication for your child is a snap, and other times, the process takes months of experimentation.

FDA-Approved Drugs: Stimulants

As mentioned before, stimulant medications have been around and have been used successfully for many decades. However, the older forms of Ritalin and Dexedrine, common medications used in the treatment of ADHD, had a number of drawbacks, including limited dosing options, shorter duration of action, and a restricted means of administration.

Over the last twenty years, there has been an explosion of ADHD medications, which include about a dozen methylphenidate-based and about a half dozen amphetamine-based formulations. In addition to offering many choices, stimulants are handy, because they don't have to be given every day. You can take the medication on Friday and skip Saturday if you need to, but in my experience, most kids do best taking the medication almost all the time.

The duration of action for many ADHD medications has expanded so that children with ADHD no longer have to go to the school nurse for a lunchtime dose of Ritalin or Dexedrine. Short-acting and immediate release drugs (Ritalin, Methylin, Focalin, Dexedrine, and Dextrostat) are still available, and these can be very handy when only three-to-four-hour coverage is desired. (Such as a midafternoon dose for homework!)

Drugs that are supposed to last five to eight hours (intermediate) include Ritalin LA, Methylin ER (Extended Release), and Adderall. In the long-acting class of medications (nine to twelve hours) there is Concerta, Focalin XR, Quillivant, Daytrana, Adderall XR, and Vyvanse.

In addition to a longer duration of action, novel delivery systems have added to the convenience of the newer stimulants. You can, for example drink the liquid Quillivant; Methylin comes in a chewable tablet; and Daytrana is available in a skin patch. For kids who have a hard time swallowing pills, Ritalin LA and Adderall XR come in beaded capsules that can be opened and sprinkled over foods like applesauce.

Potential Benefits of Stimulant Treatment

What benefits can you expect from stimulants? Changes in a child's behavior vary with the child and the drug. Anyone who has ever seen the change in the handwriting of a child with ADHD go from sloppy to neat in forty-five minutes will describe their observation with awe.

In addition to better motor coordination, better impulse control, lower emotional arousal, improved social relations, increased compliance to parental and teacher requests, reduced risk-taking, and better short-term memory can all come along for the ride.[6] Parents and teachers are often pleasantly flabbergasted by the wonderful changes in their child or student. However, these changes often only last as long as the medication does.

Potential Side Effects of Stimulant Treatment

Side effects need to be monitored, although they don't usually present an insurmountable problem. Headaches, stomachaches, and appetite reduction are common in the beginning of treatment, and these often disappear within a few days. Slight increases in heart rate and blood pressure may also occur.[7]

Sadness and irritability are also not uncommon and should be carefully examined. These two side effects account for a good deal of adolescent resistance to medication treatment. Sadness and irritability are also more common with preschoolers and with children who have autism or IQs less than 55.[8]

Oddly enough, a side effect caused by stimulant dosing that is too high is drowsiness or lethargy. Reducing the dose will usually solve the problem. This is a side effect that often occurs during the initial drug titration (adjustment) period, and it is very important for teachers to keep an eye out for it, especially in the mornings.

Stimulants may aggravate tic disorders, but these drugs do not usually create tics in kids where they had not existed before. Alternative medication choices may be discussed, but in many kids with ADHD and tics, the ADHD is by far the bigger problem, and parents may not want to forgo the powerful benefits of the stimulants when tics remain mild.

Over the long haul, there appear to be very slight deficits in height and weight resulting from stimulant treatment. Once again, a cost-benefit analysis needs to be carefully done to decide which route to go. Alternatives may include dose reduction, periodic drug holidays, or a change to nonstimulant meds. Stimulants do not increase the risk of a child later abusing drugs, but they apparently do not protect against that risk either.[9]

FDA-Approved Drugs: Nonstimulants
Strattera (Atomoxetine)

Studies support the use of Strattera for ADHD in children.[10] This drug is approved for kids six and older and also for adults with ADHD.

Strattera has a number of advantages and disadvantages. Once or twice daily dosing can produce blood levels that provide pretty much twenty-four-hour coverage, unlike the stimulants. Nice for the evening hours! The drug also has a low potential for abuse and less negative effect on height and weight.

On the other hand, Strattera has to be taken daily, and positive effects may not maximize until twelve weeks out. Positive effects on ADHD symptoms are significant, but this drug does not provide the anti-ADHD bang that most stimulants do. In order to get both twenty-four-hour effects and anti-ADHD effects, some doctors will prescribe both Strattera and a stimulant.

Kapvay (Clonidine)

Clonidine was originally a medication designed to lower blood pressure. Two studies led to the approval of Kapvay for use in ADHD treatment with kids ages six to seventeen.[11] This drug can also be used with stimulants when stimulant therapy by itself doesn't do the job. An extended-release formulation (Clon-ER) allows for twice-daily dosing.

Significant side effects, especially in the beginning of treatment, include sedation, sleepiness, and fatigue. Blood pressure should be monitored. If discontinued, this drug should be tapered down slowly.

Intuniv (Guanfacine)

Like Kapvay, Intuniv was originally designed for blood pressure treatment, and it has two controlled studies to back up its FDA approval for six- to seventeen-year-olds. Another study suggested Intuniv may help in the treatment of ODD.[12]

Intuniv allows for once-daily dosing. The drug can also be prescribed in conjunction with a stimulant when that is indicated. As with Kapvay, exercise-related side effects such as faintness or dizziness should be evaluated, and dehydration should be avoided.

Non-FDA-Approved Medications

As mentioned earlier, sometimes when children are doing an initial medication trial for ADHD, you seem to hit the miracle drug and miracle dose right away (although you really should still try a second medication just for comparison). Other times, however, it seems that all the planets and stars are aligned against you, and none of the FDA-approved drugs seem to work. You either don't get the benefits, you get prohibitive side effects, or both.

In these cases, there are still a few medications that can be considered. Although they are not FDA-approved, they still have a useful (off-label) clinical history and may be worth considering. These medications include:

- Provigil (modafinil): a nonstimulant used for narcolepsy[13]
- Wellbutrin (bupropion): a unique kind of antidepressant[14]
- tricyclic antidepressants (TCAs), such as Tofranil (imipramine) and Norpramin (desipramine): these carry cardiac risks for kids but have shown good anti-ADHD benefits as well as assistance with comorbid conditions like anxiety, depression, and tics[15]
- Clonidine: the older blood pressure medication now converted into the Kapvay formulation[16]
- Guanfacine: the older blood pressure medication now converted into the Intuniv formulation[17]

Other MTA Medication Lessons

We learned some other lessons from the MTA study (as well as from drug research in general). You should be aware of these concepts when you are designing your own treatment program.

One interesting finding was that when the combined treatment was in place (medications plus behavior management), the presence of each treatment seemed to reduce the need for the other. Parent training and good classroom management, for example, allowed medication dosages to be reduced by 20 percent or more, and conversely, the use of medication reduced the need for intensive behavior management.[18]

Another lesson had to do with unproven or non-evidence-based therapies, such as the ones discussed in chapter 10. Such therapies should either not be used or should be introduced very carefully, because they can produce side effects of their own, interfere with the more useful treatments, or use up limited resources (time and money) that could do more good elsewhere.[19] How do you evaluate new treatments? It is very telling that the only evidence-based treatments discovered so far operate at the point where performance is required of a child. At this time, anyway, we would expect—because of the nature of ADHD—that the requirement would remain in effect for any other useful treatments.

The MTA study also highlighted the fact that ADHD treatment should be tailored—if possible—to the specific needs or demands of each situation, day, and even time of day. A child, for example, might need less medication for a weekend with minimal demands for behavioral compliance and social interactions but a bit more medication for school days or for a birthday party at someone else's house. Some kids with ADHD might not need any medication at all for an all-day outing with just one parent (versus being with the entire family). Some children with ADHD might need a carefully parent-monitored homework routine (same time, same place, same procedure) after school that is combined with the use of an immediate-release, three-to-four-hour stimulant booster dose. The booster is necessitated by the fact that the long-acting morning dose of Concerta or Ritalin LA, for example, has disappeared.

> **Key Concept**
>
> ADHD treatment should be tailored to the specific needs or demands of each situation, day, and even time of day.

Discontinuing Medication Therapy

Children who benefit from ADHD medications will need to continue taking these medications for a number of years—most likely through high school and college. This idea follows logically from the fact that ADHD is not something that will be outgrown, as well as from the fact that meds do not cure the disorder—they only relieve the symptoms. Unfortunately, some children will discontinue drug therapy prematurely because their parents saw a misguided news show on TV or because Grandma read a disturbing article in a magazine and began giving Mom substantial grief about her child "taking drugs." The amount of personal, human tragedy caused by such unfortunate decisions is impossible to calculate.

A very small number of children with ADHD will be able to discontinue meds—for the right reasons—while they are still in school. How this happens, we are not sure, since ADHD is normally not outgrown or cured by treatment. Perhaps these children are extremely intelligent, have only marginal cases of ADHD, or were diagnosed very early and received the benefit of effective treatment. Perhaps, while on the medication, they also learned several new habits and compensatory skills that were powerfully reinforced.

Many professionals recommend taking a child off stimulant medication every year or so to see if she can be successful on her own. If you consider taking this step, several rules should apply to make this break as beneficial as possible and the least aggravating.

First, the periods off stimulant medication should be very short: no more than a few days to a week. Sometimes, all you need is one or two days to tell you emphatically being off the medication is not working. Don't punish the child and everyone else by keeping him off the medication longer than necessary.

Second, explain to the child what you are doing and that there is a very good possibility that he will need to continue using the medication. Sometimes, we tell children, "You'll get one vote, your teachers get one vote, and your parents get one vote." It's obvious, therefore, that the child might get outvoted! With adolescents, of course, this is a trickier process.

Third, sometimes "*accidental* medication holidays" have already told parents and teachers that the child is not ready to go off medication. An accidental medication holiday occurs when the child goes to school after forgetting to take the medication in the morning. Many parents under these circumstances are *guaranteed* to get a call from the school because the child's behavior and attention are suddenly so much worse.

Fourth, never take a break from medication in September! Never do a medication holiday in the beginning of the school year if the child was doing well with the medication at the end of the previous year. This really bad idea has ruined school years for countless children, teachers, and parents. Bad first impressions (new teacher, new classmates) can quickly become permanent! Let the child start out the new school year on the best foot, then consider taking him off medications in November or February. (Not in December, because there is too much holiday excitement.)

Medication Mistakes

Medication for ADHD is perhaps the most potent intervention we currently have. When used with home and school behavioral management, the combination provides significant relief from ADHD symptoms and impairment, helping to provide parents and their children with happier, more productive days.

In the society in which we live, however, medication for ADHD is looked at as much more controversial than it really is. So keep your head above water. Below is a list of common medication mistakes that parents should avoid. At this point in this book, I hope you can understand and explain the reasoning behind each item.

1. Inadequate prior medical histories or physical exams
2. Not trying any medication at all
3. Inadequate follow-up, both during the critical initial titration phase as well as long-term
4. Ambivalence about using drugs (mixed feelings due to poor information, for example, can cause mistakes such as underdosing with a potentially helpful medication or the discontinuation of any attempt at drug therapy after only one drug has been tried)
5. Underdosing or overdosing due to strict adherence to body-weight formulas

6. Overlooking family problems or comorbid diagnoses
7. Summertime medication holidays that ruin a child's social and family life
8. Medication holidays when a child returns to school in September
9. Stopping medication abruptly without talking to one's doctor
10. Believing that medication cannot be used when the diagnosis is ADHD-PI (most inattentive children benefit greatly from stimulants)
11. Discontinuing medication simply because a child has hit midadolescence (people can still benefit from medication at ages eighteen, thirty, or sixty-five)
12. Using only one medication when more than one would be most helpful

The Long-Term Outlook

Over the long haul, you will put a lot of effort into the treatment of your child with ADHD. While you should continue with one professional as your team coleader, other members of the group will change, such as teachers, camp counselors, and perhaps medication prescribers. Remember, though, that two things are critical for your success: continuing education about ADHD and staying in touch with your main ADHD therapist. Treatment fatigue—and even burnout—does happen, and it may result in your efforts being diverted into useless, unproven treatments or even no treatment at all. You and your child don't have to have a session with the therapist every week, but you do need to remain in contact.

Stick with it.

13

WORKING WITH
THE SCHOOL

Patricia A. Graczyk, PhD

SYMPTOMS OF ADHD ARE typically most evident in the school environment. As a result, parents of children with ADHD often need to interact with school personnel on a more frequent and intense basis than most other parents. It is important, therefore, that parents become informed of the legal and procedural options for support in their children's schools. This chapter provides a broad overview of these supports and informs parents of ways they can work with school staff to ensure that their children are provided with positive school experiences throughout their academic careers.

This chapter begins with a discussion of the steps parents can take when their child is being evaluated for ADHD and when a diagnosis of ADHD is made. Next, I discuss guidelines for effective home-school partnerships and a problem-solving process that can be used to help pinpoint a student's specific educational needs, determine and implement appropriate interventions to address those needs, and monitor the effectiveness of the interventions in addressing the identi-fied needs. A discussion of the role of support personnel and strategies for planning for transitions follows. Next, an overview of key legisla-tion that allows for the provision of specialized supports for students with ADHD who are displaying significant challenges in school will be provided. These include the Individuals with Disabilities Education Improvement Act of 2004 and Section 504 of the Rehabilitation Act of 1973 (frequently referred to as Section 504). College is discussed next, with a particular focus on ways to help ensure that a student with ADHD has a successful college experience.

When Your Child Is Being Evaluated for ADHD

By the time a child is diagnosed with ADHD, parents may have already been actively involved with their child's teacher and other school personnel. Because ADHD symptoms are typically most appar-ent within a school environment, it may even be the case that school personnel were the first to mention to parents the possibility that their child has ADHD.

Some parents prefer to conceal the fact that their child is being evaluated for ADHD from school personnel. These parents believe it is a family matter and not one for which the school should be informed. However, this point of view can actually impede the diagnosis of ADHD, because an accurate assessment of a child's school performance is a major component of the assessment process.

Typically, the clinician doing the evaluation will request a verbal or written report from the child's classroom teacher(s). As part of the evaluation, teachers are often asked to complete behavior rating scales specifically designed to provide information regarding the school difficulties most often encountered by children with ADHD. With written parent permission, most teachers are willing to provide such information and complete the necessary paperwork.

Once a Diagnosis Is Made

Once a diagnosis of ADHD is made, it is helpful to inform the school. If a trial of medication is recommended, information from the classroom teacher and school nurse is usually crucial in determining the appropriate medication and its optimal dosage.

It is a good idea for parents to provide the school with a report from their child's doctor that stipulates a diagnosis of ADHD has been made. In the report, doctors sometimes choose to include recommendations they believe would facilitate the child's school progress. It's best to give this report to the school principal (or, for older students, the child's guidance counselor) with a request that it be shared with appropriate school personnel, especially classroom teachers.

Depending on the severity of the student's needs, he or she may be eligible for a variety of educational interventions. Some students with ADHD can have their educational needs met successfully through accommodations in the regular classroom. Other students with ADHD who require special education often can be successfully maintained in the regular classroom for a significant proportion of their school day. Up to 50 percent of school-aged children and youth diagnosed with ADHD also experience other difficulties such as learning disabilities, mood disorders, or disruptive behavior that may require additional supports in school. [1]

> **Key Concept**
>
> It is a good idea for parents to provide the school with a report from their child's doctor that stipulates that a diagnosis of ADHD has been made.

Guidelines for Effective Home-School Partnerships

Overall, educators are much more knowledgeable about the needs of students with ADHD than might have been the case in the past. Nonetheless, there are several obstacles parents could face in dealing with some school personnel. Parents could, for example, underestimate or overestimate what school professionals can do. For example, a commonly held myth among parents and clinicians is that a child is automatically eligible for special education services once a clinical diagnosis of ADHD is made. (This topic will be discussed in greater detail in a later section.) Conversely, school staff could underestimate or overestimate what parents can do. The most common obstacle voiced by many parents is that they feel intimidated by school personnel. This feeling may in part be fueled by the parents' belief that school personnel are the experts and that they, as parents, have little to offer in discussing and planning their child's educational program. Unfortunately, some educators also hold the same belief, and they may convey this attitude either openly or through the manner in which they treat parents. Regardless of the circumstances, it is important for parents to take an active role in their child's education.

What, then, can parents do to ensure that their child is provided an appropriate education? First, they need to remember that they are their child's first and primary teachers. In working with school personnel, parents should present themselves as active, contributing, and essential participants in the educational decisions made for their children. Parents and school staff should work to establish and maintain a collaborative relationship based on mutual trust and respect. Both parents and school personnel should view each other as equal partners in addressing the problems a child with ADHD could face in school. Parents should also continue to educate themselves on the needs of children with ADHD (yours in particular!) so they are able to take a greater role in the decision-making process.

Problem-Solving Process

Decision-making to address the needs of a student with ADHD can be viewed as a problem-solving process. Schools frequently use this process to determine ways to help struggling students. Therefore, it is important for parents to be familiar with the steps involved in the problem-solving sequence. The following information is offered as a general framework parents can utilize in their collaborative efforts to work with school personnel to help their child in school.

The process includes four steps:

1. problem identification
2. problem analysis
3. implementing the intervention
4. evaluating the effectiveness of the intervention

To demonstrate how this process may proceed, we will take a fairly common school problem for children with ADHD, such as not completing assignments.

Step 1: Problem Identification

You may be thinking to yourself that this is an easy step, because we already know what the problem is—the student is not completing assignments. However, in this step, we need to take a general problem as stated and define it more specifically. In what class(es) is the child not completing his work? Are all his or her assignments partially done or just some of them? What kinds of assignments is he or she more likely to leave incomplete? How often does this happen? What purpose does this behavior serve?

All of these are examples of questions that may be asked to help clarify the problem as much as possible. Once there is a clear understanding of the extent and specific aspects of the problem, you then proceed to step 2.

Step 2: Problem Analysis

In this step, the team tries to determine the why. Why isn't the child completing assigned work? What are the factors that may be contributing to the problem? Is he not completing his work because he doesn't understand how to do it? He isn't using allotted time wisely? The assignment is lengthy and he is unable to attend for more than ten minutes at a time? There are too many distractions in his work area? He uses that time to socialize rather than work? At this step, you should also consider the extent to which the identified factors may be working together to cause and maintain the problem behavior.

Once the team has determined the reasons the problem is happening, then the team members need to determine what should be done to address it. This step involves generating possible strategies that align with the problem and then selecting the intervention that the team views as most beneficial to help the student. At times, school personnel will have the primary responsibility for implementing chosen strategies, but at other times, it may be the parents. For example, if a child is not completing his homework because he doesn't have a quiet place at home to study, the parents will be the ones who are responsible for finding that quiet spot and encouraging their child to use it.

In selecting interventions, it is especially important that individuals who are charged to implement interventions are, in fact, in agreement with them. After all, they are the ones who will be expected to do the work! Often, the person doing the intervention is the classroom teacher. As parents, try to be sensitive to the extra demands that children with ADHD present to their classroom teachers. Similarly, don't agree to carry out things at home for which you as a parent don't agree or cannot do.

Step 3: Implementing the Intervention

It should be made perfectly clear who will implement each of the components of the intervention. In addition, there may be other tasks that need to be carried out to complete the intervention process. These other tasks should be delineated and assigned to a team member to ensure that the chosen intervention doesn't fall between the cracks. For example, how will the team ensure that the intervention is being implemented correctly?

In our example, one way to determine whether the intervention is being implemented correctly is to develop a checklist of steps that the parent or teacher will take to help the student get the work done and then have the parent or teacher complete this checklist each day. Another way would be to observe the student during class to see if the teacher is implementing the intervention during independent seat work. If the team doesn't take steps to ensure that the intervention is being implemented properly and the student doesn't make adequate progress, it is unclear whether the lack of progress was due to the wrong intervention being implemented or because the intervention wasn't done properly.

Step 4: Evaluating the Effectiveness of the Intervention

This appraisal can be done on an informal or formal basis. Minor changes in the intervention can occur informally in order to work out the kinks as the intervention is being implemented. More formal evaluations may include progress review conferences by members of the problem-solving team. At these meetings, parents and school personnel should review what has been done, how successful it was, and the next steps to be taken. For our example, the team might compare the amount of work the student was completing before the intervention started to the amount of work the student was completing once the intervention was implemented. The difference between the two (work completed prior to the start of the intervention compared to work completed while the intervention was being implemented) would provide the team with an evaluation of the effectiveness of the intervention.

If the intervention proves successful, the team might decide to continue the intervention as is, begin to gradually fade it out to see how well the student does with fewer supports in place, or adjust it to help the student make even more progress. Should the intervention be implemented correctly but does not result in the student making adequate progress, then the team might go back to problem identification and repeat the problem-solving process until they find an intervention that works.

The Role of Support Personnel in Helping Students with ADHD

Support personnel such as school psychologists, counselors, resource teachers, school nurses, and social workers could provide supportive services to a student with ADHD. These professionals often have extensive experience with children with ADHD, and they can serve as powerful resources to students, parents, and teachers in meeting a student's educational needs. So in addition to classroom modifications or academic assistance provided by teachers, support personnel may assist in the following ways:

- provide parents with information regarding home management strategies, local parent groups, or community activities available for children with ADHD
- help the classroom teacher implement an effective classroom management program or utilize instructional practices aligned with a child's needs
- work directly with children to improve their social skills and peer relationships
- provide counseling support for children experiencing low self-esteem
- monitor the effects of medication within the school setting

Transitions

Transitions are often challenging for children with ADHD. Thus, it is important to consider ways to help them start each new school year on the right foot, and there are steps parents can take to facilitate a successful adjustment. Bottom line: you shouldn't wait until the beginning of a new school year to start planning for that year!

Instead of waiting until the start of a new school year, it is helpful to request a progress review and planning meeting toward the end of the current school year. Participants could include the child's current classroom teacher(s), the principal or guidance counselor, and other relevant staff members. At this meeting, the child's progress should be reviewed—including what strategies worked and what didn't—and both parents and school personnel should discuss what the child will need to be successful in the coming school year. The plan might include:

> **Key Concept**
> Transitions are often challenging for children with ADHD.

- a particular teacher (if there is more than one class per grade) or homeroom teacher
- a behavior management plan
- preferential seating
- a peer buddy system
- a daily assignment sheet
- additional services outside the classroom (e.g., academic support or counseling)

In most cases, once a child's new teacher (or homeroom teacher) has been named, parents should make an appointment early in the school year to initiate a working relationship. Parents can provide teachers with information regarding their child's unique needs as well as general guidelines for classroom strategies that work for students with ADHD. Parents should assure their child's new teacher that they are willing to work with him or her in meeting the needs of their child. Again, parents should acknowledge the challenges that a child with ADHD can present to a classroom teacher.

Whenever meetings are scheduled to discuss their child's educational needs, parents should make every effort to be present and actively participate in the discussion. In most cases, school personnel will attempt to accommodate parents' schedules if at all possible. It's also helpful to request that summary reports of such meetings be written and distributed to all participants. Such summaries provide a record of the issues discussed and decisions made. They also help ensure that any recommended follow-ups are implemented.

IDEA and Section 504

When ADHD significantly interferes with a student's success in school, special education or a Section 504 plan may be warranted. A discussion of each follows.

In 1975, Congress passed Public Law 94–142, or the Education for all Handicapped Children Act, 1975.[2] This important law (and its downward extension, Public Law 99–457) guaranteed that children with disabilities were entitled to a free and appropriate public education. This law also established procedural guidelines to protect the rights of children with disabilities. When 94–142 was reauthorized in 1990, it was combined with 99–457 and renamed the Individuals with Disabilities Education Act (IDEA).[3] The most recent reauthorization of IDEA occurred in 2004. In this current version of IDEA, called the Individuals with Disabilities Education Improvement Act, an even greater emphasis was placed on accountability, early intervention, and the use of research-based practices to ensure high-quality instruction for students with disabilities.[4]

Both PL 94–142 and IDEA delineate the handicapping conditions they cover. Students with ADHD who are found eligible for services or programs under IDEA are frequently served under the categories of "other health impaired (OHI)," specific learning disability, or emotional disturbance. In the IDEA Amendments of 1997, the definition of OHI was expanded to specifically include attention-deficit disorder and attention-deficit/hyperactivity disorder as two conditions that may render children eligible for special education support, *if* the condition adversely affects a student's alertness to the educational environment and their educational performance.

If students with ADHD do not qualify for support through IDEA, they could still be eligible for additional support through Section 504 of the Rehabilitation Act of 1973.[5] Under this act, a student with ADHD would be eligible for school adaptations and interventions if it is determined that ADHD substantially interfered with a major life activity, such as learning.

Both IDEA and Section 504 require a school district to conduct an evaluation to determine if a student has a handicapping condition or disability that warrants educational interventions.[6] In the 1997 reauthorization of IDEA, "parent input" was added to the list of sources from which public schools were to seek information to determine a child's eligibility for special education support. Both IDEA and Section 504 require that interventions be implemented in the "least restrictive environment" or LRE. The LRE mandate ensures that the student's educational program differs from the standard educational program only to the extent necessary to adequately meet his/her educational needs.

If a child with ADHD is found eligible for special education support through IDEA, an individualized education program (IEP) is written that includes statements of the specific difficulties the student is experiencing in school and the steps to be taken to address those difficulties. Parents are entitled to a copy of their child's IEP at no cost.[7] If a child is eligible for support through Section 504, an accommodation plan that contains similar, but not as detailed, information will be developed and implemented. Children's and parents' rights related to the child's disability are stipulated by law.[8] Many references are available that explain both students' rights and those of their parents. These can be accessed through multiple sources, such as the child's public school or school district, state and federal departments of education websites, public libraries, or organizations such as CHADD.

Although major gains have been made in home-school collaboration, there may still be times when parents and school personnel disagree about the ways to provide a child with a satisfactory educational experience. When parents have depleted all cooperative avenues, they may need to utilize the services of a parent advocate or exercise their due-process options. All states have parent advocacy groups. Parents can find this information online or through the public library.

The Big Transition: Off to College

Many students with ADHD can be successful in college, and prior planning will greatly facilitate their success. Although the average high school student may spend one to two years researching colleges and universities, college planning for students with ADHD should actually begin much sooner, i.e., by planning for their college success during their high school years.

Why so soon? For two main reasons:

1. It is through earlier school successes that a student gains the self-confidence needed to even consider attending college.

2. College acceptance and placement decisions are based on high school performance. Thus, the better a student with ADHD does in high school, the greater the likelihood he/she will attend and be successful in college.

As an entry requirement, most colleges and universities require standardized admissions tests such as the ACTs or SATs. Some students with ADHD may be eligible for accommodations such as breaks or extra time when taking these tests. Directions on how to apply for such accommodations are typically included in the application packet for these tests. Typically, high school guidance counselors and special education teachers know how to apply for these accommodations and can help answer your questions about them.

> **Key Concept**
>
> Some students with ADHD may be eligible for accommodations such as breaks or extra time when taking standardized tests.

Most universities and colleges also require documentation of a prospective student's disability and a current psychoeducational evaluation that often includes measures of intellectual or cognitive abilities and academic achievement in reading, math, and written language.[9] For example, at the University of Illinois at Champaign/Urbana, students requesting accommodations due to ADHD currently must provide such documentation as a *DSM-5* diagnosis, evidence of early and current impairment, psychological or neuropsychological assessments as needed, how ADHD impairs the students' ability to function in an academic setting, accommodations needed, and a description of ways the recommended accommodations would address the students' needs.[10]

If your child's high school has completed a recent case study, a copy of this report may be sufficient and can be sent to the college for review. If a recent evaluation isn't available or doesn't include the necessary information, parents may request that an updated psycho-educational evaluation be done by the high school. However, it is important to know that high schools are *not* mandated to conduct additional evaluations solely to provide such information to colleges or universities. Rather, many high schools honor parents' requests for such an evaluation as a courtesy to the student and family so they need not pay for a private evaluation. If the necessary paperwork isn't available through the student's high school, then the psychoeducational evaluation can be conducted by a mental health professional in the community with the appropriate training, such as a school psychologist, clinical psychologist, or pediatric neuropsychologist.

College Accommodations for Students with ADHD

All colleges and universities that receive federal funds—whether public or private—are required to offer accommodations for students with disabilities. However, the amount and comprehensiveness of this support can vary greatly from one institution to another. So it is important to investigate the extent of accommodations available at each university that your student with ADHD is considering attending.

> **Key Concept**
>
> All colleges and universities that receive federal funds are required to offer accommodations for students with disabilities.

In addition to test results, colleges often request a listing of recommended accommodations. College students with ADHD can experience difficulties with the following: organizational skills, note-taking, attending during class lectures, completing work on time, structuring their time to complete lengthy assignments such as term papers, interacting with faculty and other students, and following rules. A student with both ADHD and another condition, such as a specific learning disability, may experience additional needs in college.

Most universities and colleges provide information on their websites and in the written material they provide applicants regarding accommodations they provide for students with disabilities. The following is a list of some (but not all) such accommodations that could be available for students with ADHD:

- early registration for classes
- audio versions of textbooks
- preferential seating

- permission to record lectures to listen to later
- advanced organizers or study guides
- frequent and specific feedback and instruction
- modified assignments
- modified test-taking procedures (e.g., extra time, alternative format, quiet area, opportunities to request further clarification of instructions)
- note-taking services (e.g., obtaining copies of class notes from other students or instructors)
- tutoring services
- writing centers
- individual or group coaching
- support groups
- individual or group counseling services

Students as Self-Advocates

Finally, students with ADHD should be encouraged and taught how to advocate for themselves! Depending on their unique needs, they should be encouraged to:

- learn who and how to ask for help
- employ coping strategies and relaxation strategies when needed
- sit near the professor during class
- audiotape lectures
- use a planner or assignment book
- seek out a quiet place to study
- ask questions when they do not understand an assignment or test question
- seek out other students with similar interests to be their friends
- utilize support services offered at their college

In Conclusion

This chapter provided an overview of ways parents and school personnel can work together to help students with ADHD be successful in school. There are several other points I would like to make before ending this chapter.

Parents Can Make a Difference

With each passing year of their school careers, young people with ADHD will encounter new teachers and new challenges. Their parents will be the one consistent factor providing continuity throughout their school years. Parents need to be active and confident in their partnership with the school, whether the school is an elementary school, middle school, high school, or even college. Parents have the knowledge, experience, and concern for their children that are unique and important in helping children and young adults with ADHD be successful in school. In other words, you do indeed make a difference! And you are not alone.

School Practices Have Changed in Positive Ways

There has been a significant increase in research and practice related to helping students with ADHD. I have mentioned a number of these in previous sections. An increasing number of effective educational practices that benefit students with ADHD have been identified and implemented in schools as part of their standard practice.[11] These include the adoption of positive behavioral interventions and supports (PBIS) to help students learn and gain recognition when they behave appropriately, a focus on preventing problems and early intervention that is typically manifested through a response to intervention (RTI) or multitiered system of supports (MTSS) framework, an emphasis on promoting students' social and emotional development, and an increased appreciation for the importance of parent involvement in their child's learning. All of these initiatives provide the school context necessary for *all* students to be more successful in school, including those with ADHD.

Always Emphasize Your Child's Strengths!

In closing, there is still one very important point to make that is relevant not only to children's school careers but also to all other facets of their life. Always, always, always keep in mind your child's strengths. Children with ADHD are typically some of the most energetic, enthusiastic, alert, creative, and perceptive students we have! Although the focus of this chapter has been on ways to accommodate the challenges these children may face in school as a result of ADHD, it is important not to lose sight of the numerous talents these children have—and to help them discover new ones!

14

CLASSROOM MANAGEMENT FOR ADHD

A FEW YEARS AGO, a twelve-year-old boy came into my office during an evaluation for ADHD (which, it turned out, he did have). During this particular interview, we were discussing his feelings about school, and I had his most recent report card. It consisted of one A, one B, one C, one D, and one F. This boy was intelligent and had no learning disabilities. The amazing variability in his grades, according to him at least, was almost entirely due to his like or dislike for the teacher who had given him that grade.

My experience has been that kids with ADHD, in other words, can be notoriously teacher sensitive. If you're a teacher, it's important to realize that how you get along with these kids—your relationship with them—can have a wonderful or a devastating effect on you, the child with ADHD, and your entire class.

ADHD statistics suggest that there will be approximately two children diagnosed with ADHD in each classroom of twenty to twenty-five children.[1] In some years, of course, a teacher might get lucky and have no kids with ADHD. At other times, a teacher may have more than his share. A concentration of children with ADHD in the same class can turn the school year into a nightmare.

Even when there is only one child diagnosed with ADHD in a class, that child is very likely to take up a disproportionate amount of the teacher's time and effort, especially if that child represents the combined type of ADHD. The suggestions in this chapter are designed to keep the time and effort required to manage ADHD as manageable as possible, while still providing the necessary direction and support for the child. Assertive and reasonable management of a child with ADHD also makes the school days, weeks, and months more enjoyable and productive for all the other kids in the class.

Note: although this chapter appears to be written primarily for teachers, it's very important that parents understand it as well. Classroom behavior management is the third proven, evidence-based treatment for ADHD, and knowing how it works can assist parents in understanding what teachers are up against at school. Parents may also find some useful tools they can adapt to home!

Managing Your Own Thoughts and Feelings

The notion that a child with ADHD is a brat whose bad behavior is the result of rotten parenting puts that teacher's classroom—and the entire school year—in jeopardy.

Believe it or not, a child with ADHD will take you to task—whether you're a parent or a teacher—regarding an important segment of your own philosophy of life. In particular, you may find yourself—and your spontaneous thoughts and feelings under conditions of frustration—exposed and clearly defined along a continuum that goes from angry/judgmental at one end to understanding/helpful at the other.

Here's an example: imagine you're driving down the street on your way to work. Another driver comes out of nowhere, cuts you off, and speeds away. After getting over your fright, you might think something like "What a jerk!" and feel angry. It's what happens next that makes the difference. Some people continue with the angry thoughts, focus on them, and even feed on them. "He has no right to do that to me. There's no reason for that kind of behavior!" The angry thoughts build, and some individuals will even speed up themselves, chasing the offender to either teach him a lesson or at least give him a piece of their mind.

After recovering from the initial blast of fear and anger, other people might think, "Maybe he's heading to the emergency room with some kind of medical crisis," or "Maybe she's late for work and afraid of losing her job." As this person entertains possible reasons or motivations for the obnoxious behavior, the feeling of anger diminishes inside, and revenge is not considered as an option.

This is not a sermon; it's brutal honesty. The fact of the matter is that your thoughts, feelings, and actions are connected. Thinking "That jerk. He can't do that to me. There's no reason for that kind of behavior!" makes us angry and makes us want to strike out and defend ourselves. Thinking "He's heading to the emergency room with some kind of medical crisis" lessens anger and makes a person feel there's no need for self-defense.

While alone in your car, of course, you have the luxury of thinking whatever you want. You also don't have a reliable way of guessing what the offender's motivation was. If you don't eventually precipitate another road rage incident, it makes little difference, perhaps, what you think or do. You're by yourself, and whatever the actual motivation of the person who cut you off might have been soon becomes irrelevant.

Things are different, however, when you're in a classroom presenting a lesson to twenty-five children, and this time, it's a child with ADHD who interrupts you (again) with an impulsive and inappropriate remark. After the initial irritation, what mode are you going to get into: angry/judgmental or understanding/helpful?

Children with ADHD can force their caretakers into this dilemma many times every day. On the one hand, irritation over obnoxious behavior does not produce an incentive to be of help; rather, anger naturally inspires negative judgments and motivation toward punishment or counterattack. On the other hand, though, a teacher has the welfare of twenty-four other kids, the child with ADHD, and himself to worry about. Getting into a war with the child diagnosed with ADHD—even though it may be tempting—will do no one any good.

How does an adult make the switch—over and over again—from an angry or judgmental stance to an understanding or helpful one when attempting to handle a child with ADHD? In many ways, each of us has to come up with our own answers, but responding to that question is what this chapter is about. Don't ever kid yourself: managing a child with ADHD is hard emotional work. The very first step is to understand and to "think ADHD."

Thinking ADHD

When you reflect on it, no one, whether a teacher or a parent, should really expect "normal" behavior from a child with a special need. You don't, after all, expect a girl in a wheelchair to run like the wind. ADHD, however, is different from physical challenges in two important ways. First, with ADHD, the challenge is hidden. The child looks normal, so you tend to think, "Why on earth can't he behave like the other children?" Second, your heart goes out to the little girl in the wheelchair. You feel bad for her, and you are sympathetic. Your heart does not naturally go out to the child with ADHD who is irritating you with impulsive, inattentive, and hyperactive behavior.

"Why on earth can't he behave like the other children?" This statement is an expression of extreme frustration, but we should not treat it as a rhetorical question. Let's treat it as a real question.

The answer to the legitimate question, "Why can't he behave like the other children?" is this: the child can't behave like other children because he has ADHD, which he can't turn off at will. While a teacher's goal is to work on normalizing the child's behavior as much as possible, she must start with what she has. That means this child is the way he is.

One good way to accomplish this kind of reality check is for the teacher to make a list of ADHD symptoms and then to rate the child on each one. After a few weeks have gone by in the beginning of the year, and she has gotten to know the youngster, a teacher can do a rating of the extent to which the child shows each ADHD symptom or trait. The *DSM-5* lists (inattentive and hyperactive/impulsive) or our eight ADHD characteristics from chapter 1 might be used.

For example, here's the list one teacher made to describe nine-year-old Jeff (10 means "a lot," 5 means "about average," and 1 means "very little" compared to the child's age group):

a. inattentiveness: 9
b. impulsivity: 7
c. difficulty delaying gratification: 6
d. emotional overarousal: 7
e. hyperactivity: 6
f. noncompliance: 8
g. social problems: 9
h. disorganization: 8

This is the child the teacher will get every morning, five days a week. The rating exercise helps define the difficult job this teacher has, but any job is at least a little more tolerable when one accepts it at face value. No wishful thinking is allowed in this business.

An even better idea is for the teacher to do the symptom rating, have the parents do the same rating, and then discuss the results with the parents. This exercise helps the teacher and parents be more realistic about what to expect from this boy or girl. It also helps them sympathize with one another. This child, in other words, is capable of frustrating both teacher and parents—through no fault of anyone—in similar ways both at school and at home.

Thinking ADHD also helps to accomplish several other things. First of all, it gives the teacher a down-to-earth idea of what the behavioral repertoire of a child with ADHD really is. Second, it clarifies for the teacher that the problem is ADHD, not a lousy parent, a kid who's out to get him or her, or that the teacher is to blame. Third, thinking about ADHD this way reduces (not eliminates) anger, because it makes expectations more realistic. *Anger is always aggravated the greater the discrepancy between what you expect and what you get.*

Managing Your Feelings toward the Child

Learning to manage your own feelings toward a child with ADHD, obviously, is no easy feat. In some ways, this skill flows directly from thinking ADHD. Here's the problem in a nutshell: how do you consistently teach, care for, and offer help to a child who is obnoxious and uncooperative more often than not? No teacher wants to admit he or she doesn't like a child. Yet the fact of the matter is that there are plenty of children with ADHD who are not liked by their teachers, their therapists, and/or their parents much of the time.

As mentioned earlier, psychotherapists call a problem like this countertransference. Countertransference refers to feelings that a therapist may have toward his or her client that sometimes interfere with the therapy itself. Hostility is a common countertransference problem in many helping and caretaking relationships.

What's a teacher to do? There are no simple or easy answers, but here are a few suggestions:

> **Key Concept**
> Countertransference refers to feelings that a therapist may have toward his or her client that sometimes interfere with the therapy itself.

1. Admit the irritation to yourself (not to the child). Don't feel guilty about this anger, and don't try to cover it up with syrupy words or behavior.

2. On the other hand, don't start a war. Don't repeatedly direct spiteful—subtle or otherwise—attacks toward the child. For example, "John, did you take your medication today?" said in front of the entire class is a thinly veiled attack. So is this: "All of you who feel John is acting like a first grader, raise your hand." Revenge is a perfectly common and normal human motivation, but it can get you into a cycle of attack and counterattack. Who suffers? Among others, your entire class.

3. Adjust your expectations. If you are really mad, it's very likely that your expectations are out of whack with reality. You are out of touch with what's truly possible at this moment. Psychotherapists have to make this kind of attitude

adjustment constantly in working with their clients. What can you reasonably expect from this kid? Not from most kids, just from this one. Do the symptom ratings.

4.   Learn about ADHD. When it comes to human beings, increased knowledge about a person, his motivation, and his behavior almost always leads to less anger. Increased knowledge means being more understanding. Two key points for school personnel are these: Can you understand what it means to have a neurologically based problem with self-control? Can you take to heart the fact that ADHD is a hereditary problem that is not caused by bad parenting?

5.   Be helpful to the child with ADHD. Accept the fact that these kids need direct, frequent interventions from you. These interventions, of course, include positive reinforcement, directions, and limit setting. Remember the paradoxical-but-true old adage: if you want to get to like a difficult person, try doing him a favor. The more enterprising and energetic a teacher is in trying to solve the problems presented by a child with ADHD, the more she is going to like that child—and the higher her (the teacher's) self-esteem will be.

6.   Teaching a child with ADHD is hard enough without what we call mental "ADHD-ons." Try to avoid these common, seductive-but-mistaken notions:

   ‣ This kid is out to get me, drive me crazy, and insult me.
   ‣ This kid's behavior shows I'm not a good teacher.
   ‣ This kid's behavior proves his parents are nuts.
   ‣ This kid's behavior is deliberate and malicious.
   ‣ This kid's a brat or a jerk—or both.

   These judgmental thoughts are not only unrealistic, but they also increase anger and the impulse toward revenge. More understanding—but also more realistic—replacements go as follows:

   ‣ This kid's inattentive, impulsive, and hyperactive behavior is frequently very irritating.
   ‣ This kid's behavior taxes my abilities as a teacher.

- ADHD is not caused by bad parenting; chances are 100 percent this child aggravates his parents in the same ways he aggravates me.
- This kid's behavior is unintentional, careless, and poorly thought-out.
- I'm in the habit of thinking that obnoxious behavior proves that the perpetrator of that behavior is a jerk.

General Intervention Principles

Now that we've discussed the critical and extremely difficult issue of understanding—or attitude adjustment—it's time to discuss intervention strategies with children who have ADHD. There are hundreds of tactics, and some of the best have been developed over the years by teachers who work with students with ADHD. Different strategies work best with different teachers and different kids. It is important to keep in mind, however, that any strategy can be undermined by an underlying base of ignorance and hostility.

Dr. Russell Barkley, clinical professor of psychiatry at the Medical University of South Carolina in Charleston and the author of several books on ADHD, has proposed a number of general principles that apply to the management of difficult ADHD behavior. Several of these will be discussed here, and they apply to parenting as well as teaching. Using these principles usually means more thought and more work, but as mentioned above, kids with ADHD don't give you a lot of choice. You will react to these children—one way or another!

One of the reasons for describing these general principles before making more specific suggestions is this: many teachers are very creative at coming up with their own specific ideas if they already have some general ideas about how a task needs to be accomplished. The task here is managing inattentive, impulsive, and hyperactive behavior.

Here are Barkley's basic principles:

Immediate feedback and/or consequences. Children with ADHD learn best from feedback that comes quickly. Praise for positive behavior as well as reprimands or consequences for problem behavior should be given as soon as possible. This means just a few seconds after the behavior takes place, when possible, not minutes or hours after.

Frequent feedback. To keep them on task, children with ADHD need to receive friendly reminders and other kinds of helpful messages more frequently than adults. ADHD involves a problem with sustaining motivation, especially when feedback or reinforcement is sparse and the child sees the task as boring.

Stronger consequences. Reinforcers for children diagnosed with ADHD must be more powerful than those used with other kids. Reinforcers must have more "pull." In addition to words, for example, rewards might include tokens, points on a chart, colorful cards, or the right to engage in special activities.

Incentives before punishments. The irritating behavior of children with ADHD naturally inspires reprimands and punishments from adults. Positive reinforcement, rewards, and praise, unfortunately, will not flow as naturally. Positive consequences, however, should be used first and should also be used more often than punishments or reprimands.

Actions speak louder than words. Nagging, lecturing, prattling, and pleading don't work well, especially in the long run. We might add that these unhelpful tactics also make the adult using them more emotional. The more you talk, the more excited you get; the more excited you get, the more you talk. An overly emotional adult trying to handle an emotionally overaroused child with ADHD is not a formula for success.

Consistency. Children with ADHD do much better when there is predictability and structure in their everyday lives. These kids have a hard time handling change. If the rules—or the ways the rules are administered—are subject to adult whim or emotion, the result will be confusion and chaos.

Advance planning for problems. If you're "thinking ADHD" and have an idea what kinds of problem traits and problem situations a child is going to present, it is a good idea to plan management strategies in advance. Perhaps standardized achievement testing is coming up, or the child always has trouble with transition times during the school day. Thinking ADHD means replacing thoughts like "I hope today he behaves himself for a change" with thoughts like "What can I do to help him manage better this time?"

Reminding the child of the plan. Just because you are aware of the plan or the rules doesn't mean the child is aware of them, and as you know by now, one of the hallmarks of ADHD is a major case of forgetfulness. Don't think, "By this age, she should be able to remember…" Do think, "Kids with ADHD are running about 30 percent behind their peers in emotional and behavioral maturity, therefore…" Remind yourself to remind the child—concisely, of course—what the plan is and what the rules are.[2]

Now let's take a look at some specific suggestions for the classroom management of children with ADHD. You'll notice that these suggestions often incorporate some of the general principles just mentioned; they also represent only a few of the many intervention strategies that exist.

Behavior Management

Two basic rules apply to the classroom. First, children are in school to work and learn; there is a job to do. Second, kids' behavior should not interfere with the work and learning of others. Kids with ADHD-PI usually have trouble with the first rule; children with ADHD-C usually have trouble with both.

The instructor's first task here is to divide children's potential problem activities into three categories:

a. behavior that can be ignored (violates neither rule)
b. nondisruptive but inattentive behavior (violates only the first rule)
c. disruptive misbehavior (violates the second rule and often the first as well)

Behavior That Can Be Ignored

Children with ADHD, both combined and inattentive, will often do things that, at first glance, look like trouble but really aren't. Some of these activities are expressions of hyperactivity and restlessness, while others look like inattention but really aren't.

Manifestations of hyperactivity and restlessness include fidgeting with hands and squirming around in the chair. You can't ask a child with ADHD to sit still—that's a lost cause! But many children can—with a teacher's help—learn to express their restlessness within certain limits without violating either of the two rules mentioned above. Some children, for example, come up with some very creative body postures while they work. They may work just fine while kneeling on the chair, or they may do better reading on the floor. Some children are natural fidgeters; their hands always have to be doing something. For these kids, what some people call "legal fiddlers" can be helpful. These are objects, such as a rabbit's foot or pipe cleaner, which can be constantly fiddled with without making any noise. Gross–motor restlessness (arms and legs) can sometimes be reduced by one of the prevention tactics known as legitimate movement (see page 170).

Also in the category of ignorable behavior are postures and actions that make the child look as though she's not paying attention, when in reality, she is. Many kids with ADHD, for example, don't make good eye contact with a teacher when the teacher is talking. These kids may be looking out the window or staring at an object on the wall. Some are paying attention, and some are not. By gently asking them a question or asking them to repeat directions, a teacher can eventually learn which kind this particular child is, or the teacher can learn when this child is likely to be spacing out and when she is not.

Apparent inattentiveness can then be ignored; real inattentiveness can be dealt with using a secret signal (see next section).

Nondisruptive but Inattentive Behavior

When a child is off task but bothering no one else, a simple signal may be given by the teacher to the child. Many teachers prefer a secret signal—one that is, hopefully, known only to the teacher and the child. This maneuver is an attempt to avoid embarrassing the child and also to engage him in a kind of mutual problem-solving game. When the child is off daydreaming, for example, the teacher gets in a position to be seen and produces the signal—tugging on her ear, scratching her forehead, tapping her elbow with her finger, or whatever she and the child earlier agreed upon. A simple hand on the shoulder or finger on the child's desk can also work quite well.

Disruptive Behavior

For behavior that interferes with the work of other students, a simple signaling method (like counting, which is discussed in *1–2–3 Magic*) can be used. Verbal warnings, nonverbal signals, or counts can be given immediately after the behavior in question. After the third count, a consequence will take place. The consequence can include:

a. a brief time-out in a predetermined area of the room

b. time away: time spent in another classroom with another teacher who has agreed to cooperate

c. a response cost consequence: the student loses tokens or points that are being accumulated to "purchase" or earn special privileges or rewards

Goofing around or other violations of time-out may result in immediate withdrawal of an imminent privilege, such as free computer time, involvement of someone like a principal, and/or a notification of parents. When using any kind of counting or warning system, of course, the teacher should avoid all excess talking or lecturing and should remain as calm as possible.

After they are well into the school year, some teachers reduce the number of warnings that may be given prior to the final consequence. Instead of two warnings, children may only receive one. Eventually, kids may receive consequences for the first instance of a misbehavior when the teacher feels that the problem behavior is fairly serious or disruptive and enough time has gone by for the children to be very familiar with the rule involved.

Problem Prevention

Several tactics can go a long way toward preventing problems before they occur. These include the following.

Legitimate Movement

Allowing the child brief periods of time to move around is often a real blessing for everyone. These times can include going to the bathroom (although not nineteen times a day), sharpening a pencil, stretching, doing classroom chores, and taking special trips for the teacher down to the principal's office. Sometimes, movement can be used as a reward for good behavior, but this strategy should be used carefully, because many kids with ADHD need to move regularly—not just at special times.

Other examples of allowing for legitimate movement include the child being able to move from one desk to another to do his work. Standing work stations or the use of a podium allows some kids to get a break from sitting while they continue their work. Beanbag chairs on the floor and rocking chairs have also helped, as have exercise breaks for the whole class that involving moderate, but not frantic, movement.

Teacher-led instructional activities that require movement on the part of all students also allow the child with ADHD an opportunity to be active. Holding up yes or no response cards to answer the teacher's questions or the use of dry-erase boards can be useful.

Desk Placement

A child with ADHD usually does best when his desk is up in front of the room, fairly close to the teacher. This arrangement more closely approximates the kind of one-on-one situation in which children with ADHD perform better, and it also makes it easier for the teacher to structure work for the child, monitor progress, and provide appropriate reinforcement. If the child is facing toward the front of the room, sitting in the front also minimizes distractions; visual and associated auditory stimuli coming from the other children are behind the student with ADHD.

Be Careful with Cooperative Education or Team Learning

Many kids with ADHD don't do well when they are asked to work in small groups. Desks that are close together, for example, may mean increased distractions as well as three other youngsters within kicking distance. Some teachers, however, say that some of their children diagnosed with ADHD handle team learning well, so this is another time when gentle experimentation is needed to find out how one particular child does in this group. Many kids on medication, for example, do just fine in these situations.

Maximize the Child's Strengths

It is useful for a teacher to try to discover what this particular child is good at, whether it's math or reading or simply loving to do errands. Giving a child ample opportunity to express her strong suits, and then verbally recognizing and reinforcing her efforts increases the youngster's willingness to cooperate with other tasks as well.

Structure Is Essential

Structure means that the classroom is managed in such a way that, at any one time, each child knows what he is supposed to be doing. Children with ADHD present a challenge in this regard because they don't self-structure very well. While many children can return from recess or lunch and remember to get to work on their next assignment, a child with ADHD will return from recess or lunch and get involved with whatever comes first or whatever is most interesting. The activity chosen might be looking out the window, teasing another student, or checking out the contents of the wastebasket.

Helping the child to structure his time is aided by routine. Doing things at the same time and in the same place—as much as is reasonably possible—will help the child focus. Verbal instructions of what the agenda is before an activity are also useful. Friendly reminders during the activity also may be necessary. These reminders may take the form of praising the child with ADHD—or a child sitting near him—for staying involved with the appropriate task.

The importance of structure to the child diagnosed with ADHD has another side to it. On days when change or disruption of the usual routine is inevitable, a teacher can prepare for that fact by realizing that the strategies discussed in this chapter will need to be intensified. Such disruptive changes include field trips, visitors to the classroom, days before holidays, and standardized testing. Days when a substitute teacher is needed, of course, provide a double whammy: a different teacher is a big change to start with, and the regular teacher is unavailable to help. Different schools have different methods for dealing with these days, but lack of preparation of substitute teachers, unfortunately, remains a challenge.

Encouraging the Best Work

Here are some suggestions for helping your students with ADHD to put forth the maximum academic effort:

Clear the work area. Help the child to clear his desktop of all materials that are not part of the task at hand (with the exception of "legal fiddlers").

Divide work into small, manageable units. Some children, for example, do better when they start with a worksheet that is folded in half so they can't see the whole thing. Long-term writing assignments often give older children with ADHD (or at least their mothers) fits. Separate due dates for outline, notes, rough draft, and final copy can be very helpful.

Giving directions. When giving the instructions for an assignment, try to establish eye contact with the child diagnosed with ADHD before beginning. Use the child's name, if necessary, to keep him with you as you speak, and try to keep the directions as short as possible. Using multiple modes, such as visual and auditory, in presenting instructions or new material probably makes things a bit easier for all children.

Attention checks. Sometimes, it is helpful to see if the child has really understood the task that the teacher just described. Some of these kids have become adept at looking you right in the eye while they are paying absolutely no attention to what you are saying. If it is feasible, ask the child in a nonaccusing manner what is supposed to be done.

Doing the work. Frequent checks to ensure the work is being done are often helpful. It is certainly true that there are twenty-four other kids who also need to be checked on, but students with ADHD are the ones most likely to wander off task. Many kids with ADHD start out with a bang and then fizzle out quickly. If the child is off task, secret signals can be used to bring him back. Just like neuro-typical children, kids with ADHD do best with frequent verbal or physical reinforcement.

When the work is done. Kids with ADHD often lose their completed assignments. This unfortunate problem occurs more with homework, of course, but it can also affect work done at school. Helping the child to immediately store his work in an orderly, consistent manner is essential. Color-coded notebooks can help. Assignment sheets or notebooks for unfinished work or homework should be filled out and checked by the teacher. Even older children may need assistance in setting up these organizational systems.

Many of the suggestions above, of course, are simply part of good teaching, and these ideas may not be new. What's the point? The point is that kids with ADHD need you—and your energetic skills—more!

Dealing with Parents

Maintaining a positive and consistent relationship with the parents of a child diagnosed with ADHD is essential, although it can be very difficult. School-home communication becomes more and more important the more trouble the child is having. It is axiomatic that it is very hard—or next to impossible—to discuss serious, emotionally loaded issues with strangers. Therefore, *teacher and parents (plural if possible!) should meet before the year starts*.

Teachers need to remind themselves that these parents did not cause their child's difficult behavior by the way they raised him. In addition, mothers of kids with ADHD are the ones to whom teachers often talk more frequently, and many of these mothers will come across as angry, blaming, anxious, depressed, disorganized, and extremely intense. The internal reaction of many teachers to this presentation is something akin to "Heck, lady, if I had a mother like you, I'd be hyperactive myself!" It is important to keep in mind that this temperamental parental behavior may, in fact, reflect the exact opposite reality: Mom's upset may be a manifestation of the long-term effects of this child's behavior on her. There is a strong link, for example, between childhood behavior problems and maternal depression.

For their part, parents need to remember that the teacher has twenty-four other kids in the class to worry about; the teacher's day does not revolve around their child. Parents must also give the teacher the right or freedom to have the same negative emotional reactions to their child that they do at home. Parents cannot expect infinite patience from a teacher simply because he or she was trained to be a teacher, and when a teacher does voice her frustrations, parents should try to realize that criticism of their child is not the same as criticism of them. When teacher and parents meet, experimental and flexible thinking is needed. There are quite a few recommendations in this chapter, for example, for managing children with ADHD in the classroom. There are hundreds more to be devised and experimented with. It is obviously impossible for any teacher to apply all—or even a significant percentage—of these ideas to any one child. It is also true that not all techniques will work equally well with all children or with all teachers.

Teachers and parents, therefore, should take a provisional and pragmatic attitude toward the problem, trying to find the strategies that do the most good and that are most realistic in terms of the teacher's time, energy, and experience. The "experiment" can be accomplished in the following way:

1. The teacher sits down with the parents and asks them what strategies have worked best with their child in the past.
2. The teacher looks at the list in this chapter (or in other books) and also searches her own experience, identifying tactics that she thinks would be useful.
3. Parents and teacher agree on certain techniques. These will

be the ones tried out initially during the year. If they work, fine. If they don't, there's no sense in beating a dead horse— something else should be tried.

Medication Basics

Many teachers say that they are not physicians, do not prescribe the medication, and feel uncomfortable getting involved in this aspect of ADHD treatment. Though these thoughts are certainly understand- able, they need to be modified to some extent. A teacher's knowledge about medication and involvement in the medication adjustment process can help immensely with the overall treatment plan.

Why? For one thing, many kids with ADHD are lousy histori- ans; they have great difficulty accurately describing their past experi- ences, including their positive or negative responses to medications. For another thing, even some long-acting medications don't last much longer than the school day. They're kicking in when the child leaves for school in the morning, and they have worn off by the time the child gets home in the afternoon. So sometimes behavioral changes due to medication are there to be observed only during the school day.

What this means is that much of the time, the only reliable observer of positive and negative drug effects—who is around while the drugs are active—is the teacher. True, parents can see some effects on weekends, but that's not the same as school. For treatment to succeed, a teacher's classroom observations of a child diagnosed with ADHD on medication must be communicated to parents and doctors one way or another.

Teachers, consequently, need to know some basics about the different medications and how they work. It is very important for them to have a general idea of what positive effects might be expected from stimulants, for example, and also what some of the possible side effects might be. It is also helpful if a teacher is aware of the fact that you don't have to wait a month (with most stimulants) to determine if a drug is working; three to five days usually does the trick. Thus, if the teacher knows the child has been taking a particular dose of a certain drug for two weeks and there has been no behavior change, it's time to say something.

Some teachers (and parents) have said, "Have you ever tried to get a hold of a doctor?" True enough! If you're a teacher and you have a child in your class on ADHD medications, get a release from the parents at the beginning of the school year. Then, when you need to communicate with the prescribing doctor, send a fax or an email and copy the parents.

Teachers certainly don't prescribe medications themselves, but they can pass on critical information to parents and directly to the prescribing doctors. In doing so, they can help the child diagnosed with ADHD immeasurably. They also help make their classroom a much more positive learning environment for everyone.

15

ADHD: A LIFELONG PROPOSITION

FOR A LONG TIME, people believed that ADHD would be out-grown by the time the individual who had it was an adolescent. This idea probably came from the general observation that most hyperactive children seemed to calm down some as they got older and as their gross-motor restlessness decreased. Since the most obvious symptom of the disorder—moving around a lot—lessened, people tended to assume that the rest of the problem had gone away too.

Unfortunately, this is not the case. If current estimates are correct, 5–7 percent of children and 3–5 percent of adults have ADHD.[1] That means that about two-thirds of children with the diagnosis carry their ADHD symptoms into adulthood and also suffer the added residual problems that can arise from growing up with ADHD.

> **Key Concept**
> 5–7 percent of children and 3–5 percent of adults have ADHD.

In addition, adult ADHD is usually accompanied by other psychiatric disorders, making diagnosis more complicated. Adults with ADHD will have at least one other disorder 80 percent of the time, two other disorders at least 50 percent of the time, and three other diagnoses 33 percent of the time. These other problems include drug and alcohol abuse, depression, and anxiety.[2]

Since, by definition, ADHD involves pervasive and substantial problems with executive functioning or self-control, you would expect—especially with the added comorbidities—that in adults with ADHD, you would get sizeable impairments in many different aspects of living. Unfortunately, recent research reveals that that is exactly what happens. Adults with ADHD are:

1. twice as likely as the rest of the population to be overweight or obese[3]
2. at greater risk for coronary heart disease[4]
3. two to five times more likely to experience accidental injuries, more repeated injuries, and more severe injuries[5]
4. more likely to be poorer drivers, having more crashes, more severe crashes, more traffic violations, and more driving aggression and road rage[6]
5. more likely to have poor or failing grades and less likely to graduate college[7]
6. more likely to have been fired by their employer, to have impulsively quit a job, and to report chronic employment problems[8]
7. at greater risk for money management problems, including saving, writing bad checks, impulsive buying, exceeding credit card limits, and having utilities turned off[9]
8. more likely to have problems with marital/intimate relationships and with parenting.[10]

This, certainly, is a discouraging list, but it does not mean that all adults with ADHD are miserable. Adults with ADHD have a broad range of occupations from successful doctors, lawyers, land developers, and accountants to those who have had over twenty different low-paying jobs in their lives and are often unemployed, much like many adults across the board are.

ADHD Characteristics in Adults

The eight ADHD traits, which we described in part I, also appear in a modified form in adults. With adults, however, big differences occur in these symptom patterns because their lives have been transformed: school, for example, has been replaced by a job, and the role of being a child has been replaced by being a husband, wife, or parent. Adults have much more freedom to do what they want—for good or bad! Let's look at our list of ADHD characteristics from the adult perspective.

Inattention (Distractibility)

Adults with ADHD will still find themselves having trouble concentrating on any number of things. They may have trouble staying on task when they are at work, with the result that they do not finish as much work as they should. Distractibility can also affect adults with ADHD outside of work—they may go enthusiastically from project to project without ever finishing any one task, or they find they can't stay on top of household chores. The day is one endless series of frustrations.

Inattentiveness also frustrates adults with ADHD in social situations, where they can have considerable difficulty focusing on conversations. Some men and women with ADHD find big parties or family get-togethers frustrating because so many conversations are going on at the same time, and their mind keeps getting drawn away from the conversation they are supposed to be paying attention to. The result is frequently embarrassing when it becomes apparent to other people that the individual with ADHD has lost the train of thought or the flow of the conversation. For this reason, adults with ADHD may appear to others as if they are bored or aloof. They appear restless, do not always maintain eye contact, and sometimes interrupt or abruptly change the subject.

Impulsivity

Impulsivity is often more restrained in adults with ADHD than it is in children with ADHD. This difference may be due to the fact that by the time they are adults, these individuals may have been burned so much by past impulsive actions that they are more or less forced to exercise more self-control. (Their learning curve may be slower than average, but it's still there!)

By adulthood, many adults with ADHD are nervous about social situations for fear of what they might do or say. This discomfort may be especially strong in social situations where a man or woman with ADHD doesn't know other people well. In fact, some adults with ADHD will be quiet and appear shy when confronted with strangers. When together with familiar people or family, however, these adults often show a marked tendency to interrupt, blurt things out, talk very loudly, or even yell. Impulsivity can also raise its dangerous head when an adult with ADHD is behind the wheel of a car. Speeding, running yellow lights, and quickly becoming enraged at others' driving often make for dangerous situations.

Difficulty Delaying Gratification

Impulsivity and difficulty with delay are related problems. Impulsivity refers to action taken without thought and without waiting. Difficulty with delay is the sense of impatience and severe frustration felt internally by a person with ADHD when he is forced to pause, just sit, and think. During conversations, adults with ADHD may have an awful time waiting to express their opinion about something; they become squirmy and lose eye contact. They also may have trouble finding the patience for tedious tasks such as balancing a check book, filling out and filing a tax return, paying bills, or even reading a magazine.

Like children diagnosed with ADHD, adults with ADHD want to get these boring tasks over with as quickly as possible. This frustration and difficulty with perseverance often result in messy, unchecked, or undone work, resulting in problems that later come back to haunt the individual.

Many adults with ADHD have serious problems managing money because they spend it so quickly.[11] Since credit cards today offer the promise of never having to wait for anything, credit limits may be quickly pushed to the max. Unfortunately, spending money is sometimes seen—by people with ADHD and people without—as an antidote to boredom and other dysphoric moods.

Adults with ADHD often find that when they are inactive, they are very easily bored. This boredom can all too quickly evolve into a sense of emptiness and melancholy that is hard for them to describe but that is very painful and that they will do almost anything to avoid. Unfortunately, even though the dollars are not really available, going shopping (at the mall or on the Internet) can become a frequent—but ultimately self-destructive—exercise in financial self-medication.

Emotional Overarousal

This is one of the ADHD characteristics that is, for some reason, still conspicuously absent from the *DSM-5* list. In children with ADHD, you will recall, emotional overarousal manifested itself in the "hyper-silly" routine in groups and in ferocious fits of temper. In adults with ADHD, hyper-silly behavior in groups is much less common. Perhaps these adults have learned that this type of display doesn't go over too well with other people, or perhaps these individuals just don't feel like goofing around as much as they used to.

Temper is another story, however. I have found that adults with ADHD often continue to have temper outbursts that are about as bad (although not as frequent) as those they had as children, and these episodes can be quite intimidating to other people. Although their emotional eruptions may be more restrained in public, adults with ADHD may come across on the job as irritable or moody. At home, unfortunately, their temper may be unleashed on spouses and children. Spouses often find that they have a very hard time asserting themselves with their partner, because so many of their conversations seem to produce angry responses. Displays of temper can also be aggravated by alcohol or drug abuse. Spouses begin to feel like they are always walking on eggshells and that the moods of their mate are quite unpredictable.

In addition, a parent with ADHD may continue to show a problem with low frustration tolerance when it comes to dealing with his or her kids. Even average or typical children can be very frustrating on a regular basis. Since ADHD tends to be hereditary, adults with ADHD tend to produce children with ADHD. Thus we wind up with an adult with low frustration tolerance who has children who are unusually frustrating.

Unfortunately, this combination can result in episodes involving physical abuse. On the other hand, some parents have said that having ADHD themselves sometimes helps them understand their children diagnosed with ADHD better, because they know what the youngsters are going through and can better imagine what their children feel like inside.

People who do not have ADHD probably have no idea what kind of strain the symptom of emotional overarousal puts on the self-control of an adult with ADHD. These adults certainly do not ask that everything feel like a big deal, but it does. Neurotypical adults know what it is like to be more irritable at the end of a long day or perhaps after a few drinks, but this is an unusual experience for them, not an everyday occurrence.

For adults with ADHD, this level of emotional stimulation is a regular part of daily life. It's almost as if the same event creates in an individual with ADHD four times the amount of adrenalin that it does in someone else. It certainly is difficult to like or to understand an irritable person with a bad temper, but the old saying, "Walk a mile in my shoes," is applicable here.

Whatever underlies the problem of emotional overarousal and difficulty with emotional control may also underlie the comorbidity of adult ADHD with anxiety disorders and depressive disorders. Everyone feels anxious and depressed from time to time, but when the frequency, intensity, and duration of these feelings become excessive, anxiety or depression may be diagnosed. That is exactly what often happens in many adults with ADHD.

Hyperactivity

As they get older, most individuals with ADHD will tend to move around less. But in adults, the old gross-motor hyperactivity may be replaced by a general kind of fidgetiness or restlessness, and some adults with ADHD are still described by those familiar with them as not being able to sit still for very long. Others will continue to be hyperactive, but the hyperactivity will take a verbal form. Their speech may be rapid, nonstop, and often seems to have an anxious or driven quality to it. Individuals with ADHD may also have great difficulty stopping long enough to listen to what someone else is saying. Too often, they feel compelled to interrupt in order to make what they think is an important or critical point.

Noncompliance

As most people get older, they generally have less of a problem following rules and staying out of trouble. This positive tendency applies to adults with ADHD as well. Part of this constructive change is simply due to the fact that adults with ADHD are in fewer situations where other people are trying to tell them what to do. As parents, they may now be trying to tell their kids what to do!

Still, some studies indicate that as many as 25 percent of adults with ADHD may have a serious problem with antisocial behavior.[12] The risk of criminal or antisocial activities in adulthood, though, seems to be more related to the existence of those kinds of externalizing behaviors in adolescence than simply to the presence of ADHD.

Many adults with ADHD function well enough in the workplace because they are their own bosses. Others, however, may have quite a bit of difficulty with supervision, which tends to stir up some of the old "anti-parent" antagonisms that were experienced when they were kids. Rules and supervisors may stimulate a kind of automatic opposition; managers and bosses may be easily perceived as stupid and irrational. Remember that about half of children with ADHD also qualify for oppositional defiance (ODD).[13]

Because adults with ADHD frequently are unable to get their act together around the house and they also show great emotional lability, the spouses of these adults may sometimes feel like they have another child to deal with rather than an equal partner. However, trying to parent your spouse with ADHD is fraught with danger, because attempts at advice or correction are often met with temper outbursts.

Many spouses, therefore, simply keep their mouths shut, but inside, they feel considerable resentment toward their partner.

Social Problems

How one gets along with the rest of the human race is extremely important to anyone, and adults with ADHD are no exception. Unfortunately, I have spoken with many adults with ADHD who feel isolated and rather lonely—though this feeling may wax and wane. For these individuals, it is often hard to maintain long-lasting relationships, and by the time they are adults, some have simply quit trying. Inside, they may tend to blame everyone else for their problems, but they may also, from time to time, have the sneaking suspicion that they are the primary source of their own troubles.

At home, the temper and bossiness of an individual with ADHD can pose persistent difficulties to his or her spouse and kids. On the job, coworkers may also find the individual hard to be with due to his talkativeness, restlessness, tendency to complain, and general irritability. On the other hand, sometimes adults with ADHD are enjoyed for their lively personalities and their ability to get a discussion—or a party—going, and this skill can help their social lives considerably.

Disorganization

Many adults with ADHD have trouble juggling the different aspects of their lives. They can have trouble with dates, times, and appointments, and—as with children with ADHD—their memory can be erratic. The homes of men and women with ADHD are sometimes monuments to the tendency to start and not finish things. The bathroom upstairs has been torn up for the last six months, there are still paint cans on the floor of the kids' half-painted bedroom, and the car had to be parked outside all winter again because the garage cleaning project never got done.

On the job, adults with ADHD can have difficulty staying with a task, especially if they see it as boring and if it is entirely up to them to keep at it. Because adults with ADHD are easily bored, they tend to avoid tasks that they feel are uninteresting or obnoxious, such as anything that feels like school. They also gravitate toward the easiest or most interesting thing to do at the time. The problem with this way of operating is that the job chosen may not be the one that most needs to be done at that moment.

An adult with ADHD may also feel like he is a born procrastinator. At work, such procrastination may get many adults with ADHD into significant trouble. Over time, the quantity of undone, boring tasks builds up. The employee begins to feel more and more embarrassed about the incomplete jobs, but he still can't bring himself to face the unpleasantness. Then he is confronted by an angry supervisor who has finally discovered the gap in the work, but the individual with ADHD cannot provide a reasonable explanation for what happened.

Many men and women with ADHD, of course, handle life very well. Most will be married, have jobs, and be self-supporting. Some adults with ADHD—especially if they are bright, energetic, and have good social skills—can conquer the world. With good brain power and the ability to get along with others, these individuals use their extra ADHD energy to good advantage. Though ADHD may continue to add some rough edges to their existence, these men and women become outstanding achievers.

16

DIAGNOSIS OF ADULT ADHD

OUR ESTIMATE OF THE prevalence of adult ADHD is 3–5 percent.[1] Let's go with 4 percent for a second. If there are about 324 million people in this country, that means we have around 13 million adults with ADHD. That's a lot of people! Many mental health professionals who work with ADHD wonder where all these people are hiding out.

How do adults with ADHD get into treatment? Obviously, most of them don't. Undoubtedly, many adults avoid treatment because they feel that, as kids, they were dragged to every doctor in town, and they're sick of doing that. Now that the decision is up to them, they don't especially care to see another mental health professional or another physician to discuss their inadequacies.

On the other hand, there are many individuals with ADHD who stick with treatment through their childhood, adolescent, and adult years. They have realized that this perseverance makes a big difference in their lives and that it also makes those around them a lot happier. As one adult with ADHD put it, "I'd rather be happy than go around pretending I'm perfect and shooting myself in the foot all the time."

What about men and women with ADHD who were never diagnosed as children or teenagers? It is very common for adults to seek treatment for themselves after their child has been successfully diagnosed with ADHD and treated. In the course of their son's or daughter's evaluation and therapy, these parents learned that ADHD is usually hereditary and that it is often not outgrown When discussing the developmental histories of their children—and their own during their child's evaluation—many adults can't help but see the remarkable similarities of their own pasts to those of their kids. During the evaluation of one kindergartner who seemed to be driven by a motor, the boy's father recalled that when he was in kindergarten, his teacher had tied him (the father) to a chair to restrict his activities!

Involvement in support groups for parents who have children with ADHD may also help to reinforce the idea that residual—or adult—ADHD exists. During such meetings, parents may meet other parents whose situations are similar to their own, and parents may start wondering, "What about me?"

After doing a fair amount of soul searching, many adults will come into the office, convinced they have ADHD. Some of these people are correct, although there may be other diagnoses as well. However, a competent therapist will carefully check the available information and conduct an evaluation similar to what would be done with a child. In some cases, adults consult more than one therapist for a diagnosis. For example, some people who were diagnosed in the past with bipolar disorder, a chemical dependency, or schizophrenia may consider the diagnosis of ADHD to be more benign and therefore more desirable than their other diagnoses. Motivation for treatment can also come from other sources. A frustrated wife, for example, may know she has a child with ADHD, but she may be convinced her husband has the condition too. Many women try to encourage their husbands to do something about the possible problem. Some are successful. Other times, the other person gets defensive, and arguments result, which reduces motivation for treatment. It certainly is no help if one feels that seeking an evaluation for ADHD is like eating crow.

Diagnostic Criteria for Adult ADHD

The inattentive and hyperactive/impulsive lists from *DSM-5* are also used in diagnosing adults with ADHD. The problem with this is that for many adults, their symptoms may not be as intense as when they were children, but they don't usually go away with age. Generally, inattentive symptoms are more durable than hyperactive/impulsive symptoms.

Two results may follow from the mellowing of symptoms. First, many adults who are still truly troubled by ADHD may not qualify for six of the nine symptoms on either or both lists. The result of this first consequence is that people who would have been characterized as having true ADHD-C will begin to appear—according to *DSM-5*—as though they have ADHD-PI.[2] They will meet at least six of the nine inattentive criteria but will not fit more than six hyperactive/impulsive traits. In response to this concern, *DSM-5* lowered the cutoff score required for adults on both lists from six to five. Some people think the score could even go down to four for adults without sacrificing diagnostic accuracy.

Since ADHD has so many comorbidities, one of the most helpful considerations for the evaluator is the chronic nature of the ADHD symptoms. To qualify as an adult with ADHD, you must have had ADHD as a child (whether diagnosed or not), with symptom onset before age twelve. ADHD does not just start up suddenly when you hit age thirty-five; there must be evidence of chronic, ADHD-based impairment throughout your life.

The diagnosis of adult ADHD requires several steps that are similar to those included in the evaluation of a child, but there are important differences. The steps for evaluating adults include:

1. self-reports of the adults themselves regarding presenting complaints
2. developmental history, including family history, educational, workplace, and social functioning, and medical and psychiatric history
3. structured interviews, rating scales, and questionnaires

4. observations of office behavior
5. interviews with spouses, parents, or others who know the adult being evaluated
6. other information

Adult Self-Reports

Therapists who work with ADHD in adults are very familiar with the impatient phone call from someone who says, "I have adult ADHD, and I'm ready to do something about it." The message is, "Let's get going. I'm frustrated and in pain! Why waste any more time? I know what the problem is!" Sometimes, it takes quite a bit of effort to persuade an ADHD candidate to submit to the entire process of evaluation, which takes three or four sessions plus some homework.

Just like their younger counterparts, adults with ADHD are not always good historians when it comes to describing presenting complaints or providing a developmental history. Though they may be able to describe the things that currently cause them emotional pain, they may minimize problems in which their angry, intrusive, or hyperactive behavior causes trouble for others. You will also recall the positive illusory bias that is often characteristic of kids with ADHD. A poor memory can also make sifting through past years a formidable task for both client and evaluator. Disorganized thinking and the patient's likely tendency to jump from topic to topic also put pressure on a mental health professional to structure the interview so that the necessary information is retrieved.

What problems do many adults describe when they come in for evaluation? As I mentioned, some start by telling the therapist or evaluator what they think their diagnosis is. Other adults describe presenting complaints that involve mood (depression and/or anxiety), job concerns, and marital dissatisfaction. Both men and women can report the pervasive feelings of melancholy and dissatisfaction with life that accompany depression or the agitation and discomfort of anxiety. Women are often more honest in describing the low self-esteem that accompanies mood problems, while men may vacillate between blaming everyone else for their troubles and being able to describe their own shortcomings.

Men mention job concerns more often than women. Their concerns include difficulty concentrating, procrastination, trouble getting started, poor organizational skills, and difficulty getting along with others. Add all these up, and the adult often feels that he isn't progressing as quickly as he would like at his place of work. These problems have been brought up by supervisors in periodic performance appraisals, often leaving a residue of intense anger as well as nagging self-doubt.

Marital problems are usually brought up more often by women. Since women are often affected by ADHD-PI, they may report that their husband criticizes them for the disorganization of the household. These women also feel that, in discussions and arguments with their spouses, they cannot hold their own; they get mixed up, flustered easily, and have trouble expressing themselves. This confusion is infuriating, because it adds to the conviction of their spouse that he was correct in the first place.

In marriages where one spouse turns out to have an adult version of ADHD-C, the non-ADHD spouses will also have a great deal of difficulty asserting themselves with a person who doesn't listen well, interrupts frequently, and often has a ferocious temper.

Some adults with ADHD present complaints that are less specific and also more confusing. Their complaints can include not being in a very good mood much of the time and vague hints regarding low self-esteem. One theme that often jumps out is how aggravating other people are—from family members to friends, coworkers, and even the government. Other less well-defined complaints may have to do with not feeling well-organized, difficulty persevering with a wide range of tasks, and a sense of memory loss or confusion.

Structured Interviews, Questionnaires, and Rating Scales

The good news about structured interviews, questionnaires, and rating scales is that they can help organize the evaluation process so that it is more reliable and valid. Structured interviews help the evaluator assist the person being evaluated to stay on task. Questionnaires and rating scales, which can be mailed out before the first office visit, give the adult time to think and reflect about their possible diagnosis. The bad news, however, is that a paper- and-pencil task that requires reflection is generally not the kind of job that someone with ADHD enjoys.

Several instruments are helpful for taking a closer look at presenting complaints and comorbidity. The Structured Clinical Interview (SCID) can take the interviewer and client through the *DSM* diagnoses in a way similar to what the DISC does with parents of kids. The Symptom Checklist 90–Revised (SCL-90), and the Personal Problems Checklist for Adults are broad-band scales that look at a wider range of symptoms, such as anxiety, depression, hostility, and obsessive-compulsive traits.

The daunting task of completing an accurate history can be aided by using the Wender Adult Questionnaire-Childhood Characteristics Scale (AQCC) or Goldstein and Goldstein's Childhood History Form. In *Attention-Deficit/Hyperactivity Disorder: A Clinical Workbook*, Barkley and Murphy also provide developmental history, health history, employment history, and social history forms that can be duplicated at no charge. Some professionals ask that these forms be completed not only by the person being evaluated, but also by a spouse, friend, or parent.

ADHD-specific (narrow-band) instruments include the ADHD Symptom Rating Scale, which is from *DSM-IV* but can still be used. This scale allows each of the possible eighteen ADHD symptoms (nine inattentive, nine hyperactive/impulsive) to be rated for severity on a four-point scale, rather than the all-or-nothing format that is usually employed with the *DSM-5* criteria. Clients as well as spouses can fill out the form to describe an individual's current functioning; clients and parent(s) can fill out the form to describe the individuals functioning as a child. The Attention Deficit Disorder Evaluation Scale (ADDES-4) also has adult versions that include evaluations of social life and employment.[3]

Other narrow-band instruments can help the evaluator take and look at specific non-ADHD areas. These scales include Locke-Wallace Marital Adjustment Scale, the Hamilton Anxiety and Depression Scales, and the Michigan Alcohol Screening Test.*

Office Behavior

While 80 percent of children with ADHD will sit still in a doctor's office because it is new and intimidating and not show their ADHD symptoms during the visit, I have found that the same is not true of adults.[4] The office behavior of adults with ADHD will frequently reveal a number of characteristics that are related to or the result of attention-deficit/ hyperactivity disorder. Rapid speech is very common, and the steady flow of ideas may almost overwhelm the interviewer. However, the ideas are often not very well organized. The adult may shift from one story to another, and the listener may struggle to try to figure out what the point of a particular story is. In my experience, an adult with ADHD may seem quite anxious, restless, and driven, sometimes presenting an almost haunted look, as if he can't escape some dark cloud that follows him everywhere. Eye contact is often broken, and the individual will sometimes appear as if he is lost in thought, pausing for a few seconds and staring off into the room.

One of the most common occurrences in interviews with adults

---

* The Locke & Wallace Marital Adjustment Test (MAT) measures marital satisfaction. Often considered the gold standard of public domain marital satisfaction measures, the scale focuses on issues such as involvement in joint activities, demonstration of affection, frequency of marital complaints, level of loneliness and well-being, and partner agreement on significant issues.

 The Hamilton Anxiety Rating Scale (HAM-A) is a psychological questionnaire used by clinicians to rate the severity of a patient's anxiety, and it was one of the first anxiety rating scales to be published. Originally designed by Max Hamilton in 1959, the HAM-A remains widely used. For clinical purposes and for the purposes of this scale, only severe anxiety is at issue. The Hamilton Depression Rating Scale (HAM-D) is a way of determining a patient's level of depression before, during, and after treatment. It should be administered by a clinician experienced in working with psychiatric patients.

 One of the most widely used measures for assessing alcohol abuse, the Michigan Alcohol Screening Test (MAST) is a self-administered questionnaire designed to provide a rapid and effective screening for lifetime alcohol-related problems and alcoholism. The MAST has been productively used in a variety of settings with varied populations.

is their tendency to interrupt the interviewer. This trait takes some getting used to! The symptoms of difficulty delaying gratification and impulsivity seem to operate here. The person suddenly gets a good idea and simply can't wait to share it, no matter what the interviewer is saying at the moment. Many adults with ADHD are aware of this tendency and tease themselves about it from time to time, although that insight doesn't necessarily cut down its frequency.

The overall mood of an adult with ADHD may alternate between sadness, excitement, and irritation. So many things seem to bother these men and women. Then, it seems, the emotional aftermath of this aggravation is sadness, brief depressive episodes, and a feeling that life is generally very frustrating and discouraging. Though adults with ADHD often blame their troubles on the behavior of other people, after they become comfortable with the interviewer, they can begin to get in touch with and express doubts about themselves.

Find Mom! Interviews with Spouses, Parents, and Others

It is very important for the therapist or evaluator to talk with other people who know the adult they're evaluating. Just like kids with ADHD, adults with ADHD are not always good historians, and they often don't remember a lot of important pieces of information. In addition, adults with ADHD are not always objective, and they may show a distinct tendency to minimize certain aspects of their problems. While they might be quite candid, for example, when discussing their concentration difficulties, they may omit a lot when it comes to how they express their hostility at home with the family.

The client's mother can be an invaluable source of information if she is still alive, and spouses and partners should definitely be included in the evaluation too. One reason for involving the spouse, of course, is that this person will be not only helpful for information but also necessary as treatment progresses. The spouse should be seen separately, at least part of the time, so he or she can talk freely. Many times, the stress the spouse or significant other feels is painfully obvious, and there is some relief in being able to vent about his or her frustrations. Spouses describe issues such as someone who often swings between anger and depression; difficulty talking to the spouse, who seems to take everything as a criticism; intolerance of the children; arbitrary and inconsistent discipline; excessive use of alcohol; chaotic spending and money management; and a host of unfinished projects around the house. Some spouses describe a feeling of guilt because they avoid their husband or wife and feel relieved when their partner is not around.

Other Information

When evaluating adults for ADHD, much of the same information is helpful that is useful in diagnosing children. The problem is much of that information is not as readily available. School records, such as report cards, achievement tests, and reports describing special education interventions are extremely helpful to the evaluator. They can also be quite interesting to the person being evaluated, as it can stimulate other important—and sometimes painful—memories.

If records of psychological testing can be found, these reports can be very helpful. Most clients are very curious about test data (such as their IQ score) and appreciate having it explained to them. If psychological testing was never done, it is sometimes a good idea to consider something like an adult IQ test and some achievement tests that have adult norms. Keep in mind that if medication is to be considered later as a possible treatment alternative, the choice of a medication and its titration should probably be done before the psychological testing is done, so as to get the most accurate results.

Performance appraisals from work, in the form of evaluation scales and/or written narratives, can often provide a more accurate picture of an individual's strengths and weaknesses on the job. Perhaps equally important is the adult's attitude toward and feelings about these appraisals. What feedback from his supervisors does he agree with, and what does he see differently? How well has the individual liked his immediate superiors? Some adults who come in for an evaluation are willing to have a mental health professional contact their current boss or supervisor, but many, of course, do not wish to reveal to anyone at work that they are going to see a therapist.

A health history is an important part of the ADHD evaluation. Sometimes, a physical exam is needed as well. Gathering this information is probably even more important with adults, because adults have had a greater period of time in which to incur physical problems, may have a greater range of possible problems, and may also have had some difficulties with drug or alcohol misuse. Certain physical conditions may produce symptoms that mimic ADHD. These conditions include diabetes, cardiac difficulties, thyroid dysfunction, and chronic pain. As mentioned earlier, the chronic nature of ADHD and its early onset often help distinguish it from other physical and emotional problems.

> **Key Concept**
> A health history is an important part of the ADHD evaluation.

Diagnosis Shock

For the adults who are diagnosed as having ADHD, the discovery that they have a particular problem is something that has a number of positive as well as negative sides to it. Many adults with ADHD are in something of a state of shock for a while as the diagnosis sinks in. *You mean it has a name? There is, in a sense, something inside me—a diagnosable disorder—that has been causing all this trouble. And this thing is not the same as my inner self or the "real me."*

On the positive side, therefore, the diagnosis brings with it the idea that *all the problems may not have been my fault. It wasn't "just me" that was doing it. And all the people who criticized me in the past didn't know the whole story.* The individual may also begin to feel that he is not alone. Many other people suffer from the same problem, and comparing notes with other adults with ADHD can often be a beneficial experience.

Also on the positive side is the feeling that perhaps something can be done about the problem. *I don't have to be this way all the time.* One of the most dramatic examples of this realization for many people is their first experience with medication. Some men and women with ADHD have experimented with their children's stimulant medications; others have waited for their own prescriptions. For those who respond well to medication, the experience often feels like some kind of religious awakening. On medication, adults with ADHD can pay attention to details that were previously unrecognized. With the help of drug treatment, these men and women may suddenly be able to sit still during a conversation and really listen to what someone else is saying without feeling the restless urgency to either speak or leave. Daily activities can be organized better, and work becomes more productive.

Many adults with ADHD will take antidepressant medication, either in addition to (in the case of comorbid disorders) or instead of stimulants. Although the effects of these drugs can take several weeks to kick in, a positive response to antidepressants can also be an enlightening experience. Some people say that they never knew how depressed they were until they started feeling better; that lousy feeling had just been taken for granted all these years.

The diagnosis of ADHD, however, may also have a negative side. It can bring a sense of many wasted years. *If only I had known, I could have been saved a lot of trouble.* The diagnosis can also generate considerable anger toward those who didn't do anything constructive about the problem in past years—especially parents. Even though it does not always make sense, this resentment can still be strong, especially when the ADHD trait of emotional overarousal adds its power to the feeling.

Following the diagnosis, as a person learns more and more about ADHD, other negative issues can arise. Dramatic initial responses to medications, for example, can generate hopes for a permanent cure or permanently altered state of being. Over time, however, the realization hits that ADHD is not curable. In addition, the effects of stimulant medications only last for a short period of time, and most people can't take them in the evening due to the possibility of insomnia. Some adults also find—as do some children—that the

ADHD symptom of disorganization makes it hard for them to stick to a regular medication regime.

There can be other downsides. Medications can involve considerable expense. For many people, the idea of taking pills for the rest of their lives is also not very appealing. Perhaps it's the old American tradition of "rugged individualism" that makes the idea of chemical assistance for mood or behavior unsavory. By and large, though, a valid diagnosis of ADHD offers the possibility for new ways of looking at life, much greater personal and professional success, and more satisfying relationships with other people.

17

TREATMENT FOR ADULTS WITH ADHD

FOR THE THERAPISTS TRYING to treat them, adults with ADHD can be among the most enjoyable and rewarding of clients— and the most frustrating. This is a paradox their friends and family can relate to as well. Since they are no longer being dragged into treatment by their parents, adults diagnosed with ADHD also have a choice about whether to pursue counseling and medication or whether to try to manage their disorder on their own.

ADHD treatment for adults is in some ways similar to treatment for children with ADHD and their parents. Education about ADHD and about issues like medication, for example, can be quite helpful. But there are some important, positive differences when it comes to treating ADHD in adults. Because adults come in for treatment of their own volition (whereas the children do not), their voluntary participation is likely to make efforts such as counseling, social skills training, and self-control training more productive. Adults can also make more choices about treatment alternatives depending upon the kinds of work, social involvement, education, and recreation they want to pursue.

Treatment of ADHD in adults is a relatively new phenomenon, and there is a lot more that needs to be learned about it. In dealing with adults with ADHD, many therapists do their best by making educated guesses based upon what is known about counseling and psychotherapy in general and also based upon what is known about medication treatment of children.

But adults with ADHD are more complex and have more comorbid conditions to consider, and the fact that they can make the decision to pursue treatment can definitely be a mixed blessing. ADHD is still largely an externalizing disorder, and many adults with ADHD are more comfortable blaming others for their problems and not as good at taking responsibility for their own behavior. In a sense, though, once there is an ADHD diagnosis, the ADHD can be viewed as the culprit. Today, I have seen more and more adults with ADHD are being treated and more research is being done on what works.

Education about ADHD

Adults must be educated about ADHD just as parents and sometimes children are, but adults diagnosed with ADHD are usually more interested than little kids are in learning about the disorder and how it affects them. Today, a good deal of educational material—in the form of books, online resources (chadd.org and add.org), audios, videos, newsletters, and support groups—is available. Many adults with ADHD prefer to learn by means of videos or discussions with other people. They are interested in learning about the basic symptoms of ADHD and then using this knowledge to shed light on their own past and present behavior.

Education about ADHD is also the beginning of counseling. The very fact that there is a hereditary condition known as attention-deficit/hyperactivity disorder and that it produces identifiable effects in one's life can be the basis of a restructuring of a person's view of herself. As the authors Kate Kelley and Peggy Ramundo have said, an adult with ADHD may begin to realize that she is not "stupid, lazy, or crazy."[1] As everyone who has ever gone through the process knows, however, old, self-critical messages die a very slow death. The job of reeducation needs to be constant—and probably lifelong.

Seeing oneself differently also means self-esteem can change and a new kind of self—and a new life—may be possible. *If I'm not as incompetent as I always thought I was, who am I really? What unrealized potential do I have?* These thoughts are exciting, and they can be the basis for legitimate hope that life can actually improve. *Maybe I can get along with other people better. Perhaps I can do my job differently. Maybe I can even go back to school and consider the possibility of a different kind of work.*

The overall treatment model for adults is also similar to that for children, but now the team is smaller. The core team is the adult client with ADHD, the main therapist, and a doctor who initially prescribes the medication and then checks in regularly. There will be an initial period of a few months for evaluation, definition of the treatment plan, and medication titration. Then weekly visits may follow for a few more months or longer, after which the sessions are gradually spaced out more and more as things settle down and success in a new life is achieved.

Medication

Some of the medications available for children with ADHD have been used successfully with adults with ADHD. At the present time, two kinds of extended-release stimulants (amphetamine and methylphenidate) and one nonstimulant (atomoxetine) have been approved by the FDA for adult treatment.[2]

While the stimulants have been shown to help with adult ADHD, the benefits may not be quite as robust as they are with children. In addition, bodyweight formulas for estimating therapeutic dosages for children should not be used with adults, as their metabolic rate is likely to be very different from that of kids.

The stimulant medications, however, seem to be fairly well tolerated by adults. Side effects similar to those common in pediatric situations can occur. (See page 135 for information on side effects.)

However, adults must be carefully educated on how these medications may affect their lives. Stimulants plus coffee or nicotine (or both!), for example, may produce an unpleasant sense of overstimulation. Medication can also affect sleep schedules, and it can change a person's reaction to alcohol. It is important for adults to understand and accept that stimulant meds do not cure ADHD. Adults need to pay careful attention to exactly how long the benefits of the medications last and then make appropriate adjustments.

As it does with kids, atomoxetine (Strattera) offers the possibility of more consistent, twenty-four-hour blood levels, although it usually does not provide the anti-ADHD power of methylphenidate or amphetamine. Originally designed as an antidepressant, Strattera may also have some added benefits for a patient when comorbid conditions such as anxiety or depression are present. This drug has little risk for abuse, so it may be useful where adult ADHD exists with substance abuse.

The research is still out regarding adult ADHD treatment using some of the other drugs that have been successfully used with children.[3] Because of concerns about sedation and low blood pressure, little has been done with Intuniv and Kapvay. The typically unpleasant side effect profiles of the tricyclic antidepressants (Norpramin, Tofranil) have not encouraged their use with adults, especially since the advent of atomoxetine. Not much has been done with Provigil for adults, though some experts still believe the drug has promise.

The antidepressant Wellbutrin (bupropion) has shown some usefulness in treating ADHD symptoms in some limited investigations. Some clinicians have had the experience of an adult with ADHD saying what a wonderful boost they got in their ability to concentrate when they took the drug Zyban (also bupropion) to help with smoking cessation. A pleasant surprise to all! Bupropion may also help with ADHD and comorbid depression or substance abuse. Side effects include insomnia, nervousness, and possibly seizures.

Selective norepinephrine reuptake inhibitors (SNRIs) and selective serotonin reuptake inhibitors (SSRIs) have traditionally not been seen as effective for ADHD in adults or children. These drugs do not alter inattention, impulsivity, or hyperactivity. However, they do help with the comorbid conditions of anxiety and depression.

This leads to an interesting issue. Spouses of adults with ADHD frequently report that their partner with ADHD is "so much easier to live with," "less irritable," or "more mellow" when also taking an SSRI or SNRI. This may mean the changes are due to the SSRIs' having an effect on the mood disorders that often accompany ADHD. On the other hand, if you consider emotional overarousal or dysregulation to be a primary symptom of ADHD, these antidepressants could be said to alter ADHD symptoms directly.

Maybe that's why many adults with ADHD find that the best medication regime for them involves using a stimulant and an antidepressant in combination. The stimulants help best with the core ADHD symptoms, and longer-acting ones—although not twenty-four-hour—are now available. SNRI and SSRI antidepressants may not help with inattention, impulsivity, and hyperactivity, but they do help with what you might call emotional temperament—and their effects can last all day long. With a stimulant and an antidepressant, therefore, an adult diagnosed with ADHD may achieve a concentration benefit during the day, when it is most needed (at work), and may also maintain a kind of temperamental mellowing effect during the evening while at home with family or out with friends.

When it comes to medication treatment, one important rule applies to both children and adults: the principle of individual differences. Medication must be carefully adjusted, and the process frequently involves trial-and-error learning. What is best for one individual, in terms of both medication type as well as dose, may be quite different from what works for someone else.

Counseling

As we saw before, education about ADHD is the necessary beginning of individual counseling. Education about ADHD provides both bad news and good news. On the bad side, a therapist may need to assist an individual with ADHD in expressing his dismay and resentment for having ADHD symptoms. "I'm sorry you're stuck with ADHD, but here's what we can do about it." That's part of the good news; something can now be done about this problem.

ADHD symptoms may explain present and past behavior, but they are not an excuse. Part of the therapist's job is to help an adult with ADHD take responsibility for being the way he is and deal with it. Accepting the fact of emotional overarousal in one's personality, for example, is not to be taken as license to berate or abuse one's spouse or children.

Individual counseling can also provide realistic moral support. It can help adults with ADHD come to a more accurate sense of self-esteem, an aspect of their existence which has usually taken quite a pounding over the years. Many adults with ADHD, for example, have an excellent sense of humor; amusing anecdotes about forgetfulness and disorganization are now plentiful. Individuals with ADHD may find it healthy to take themselves with a few grains of salt, while at the same time working hard to improve their overall effectiveness.

Marital counseling is often helpful with adults diagnosed with ADHD and their spouses. Husbands' and wives' tales about years of frustration should be listened to (although not beaten to death), and something should be done to try to prevent the future from being as difficult as the past. Since the non-ADHD spouse has often been the chronic underdog in a relationship, a therapist can help a couple come up with a more democratic way of dealing with each other. The entire focus of counseling should not just be on ADHD, however, since the individual with ADHD will also have legitimate gripes about his or her partner that need to be addressed. Part of the focus in counseling should be on helping the couple to have fun again—something that people with ADHD are usually very good at!

Periodic family counseling can assist children and parents in dealing with the usual problems that come with daily living, as well as those that are related to ADHD. It is quite common for parents with ADHD to have kids with ADHD, and this unfortunate combination can make things very difficult around the house. When dealing with the kids, an adult with ADHD and spouse will find it helpful to learn some specific parenting strategies, such as counting, bonding, and positive reinforcement, rather than just shooting from the hip when problems come up with their children.

Self-Control and Social Skills

Individual counseling can also be the forum where someone with ADHD learns to develop his or her organizational skills. Keeping a daily planner—electronic or paper—where everything is written down can be extremely useful. The next step is developing tactics that will help the adult with ADHD not misplace their planner! Also useful can be the development of memory-jogging techniques for taking medication, the use of computers, phones, or tablets to aid in planning and completing daily tasks, and having someone teach the mechanics of balancing the checkbook and filling out income tax returns.

For adults, social skills training often takes place in the context of individual counseling. Therapists working with clients with ADHD find it a refreshing change to work with an adult who wants to change his or her ways of relating to other people, rather than with a child diagnosed with ADHD who has difficulty understanding how his behavior causes social issues. Compared to children, adults with ADHD also have more motivation to generalize their learning from the therapist's office to the real world, and many are delighted with the benefits of their efforts.

Medication can play a big role in effecting social change. Listening skills, for example, are often enhanced tremendously by stimulant medications prescribed in conjunction with counseling. Antidepressants, as just discussed, can also have a kind of calming effect that reduces the restlessness and fidgetiness that children, spouses, and coworkers find so irritating.

More and more groups for adults with ADHD are available these days. These groups include support group meetings that may take place monthly, as well as more intensive experiences in weekly groups.

Being in a small room with seven other adults with ADHD for an hour and a half can be a trying experience, but it can help people get a perspective on the disorder and realize they are not alone.

Although it does not quite fall into the category of individual counseling, a newer strategy for helping adults with ADHD is known as coaching. The coach helps encourage, support, organize, and direct the individual with ADHD, but the contacts are usually much more frequent than those involved in counseling. Instead of talking once a week or less, the coach and client communicate a number of times per week via phone, voice mail, texting, or e-mail. Sometimes, the contacts are daily, but they are of shorter duration than counseling sessions—perhaps ten or fifteen minutes. This frequency of contact can be very useful, and it is an attempt to respond to the basic ADHD problem of sustaining motivation over time.

Coaching is intended to be present-oriented, practical, and task- or goal-directed. The coach hopes to provide some friendly account-ability for the adult diagnosed with ADHD to help him stay on task, accomplish his goals, and get more out of life. Coaches who work with ADHD, of course, need to be very familiar with the problem (many coaches have ADHD themselves). The coaching movement has been building up steam recently, but there is not a lot of good research yet on its effectiveness.

On the Job

For most adults with ADHD, the curse of school is replaced by the world of work. Unfortunately, like the previous academic setting, the work world may turn out to be no picnic either. Repetitive tasks, annoying coworkers, and bothersome superiors can make the days seem endless for some people.

With the help of a sympathetic counselor, however, adults with ADHD can begin to sort out how much of the problem is the job and how much is them. In the big, bad world, there certainly are plenty of boring jobs, irritating associates, and incompetent supervisors! In counseling, an adult with ADHD can take a long look at several questions: Is this the job for me? Do I have any choice? Is this the job for me if it could be altered in some ways? Should I look for something else to do? Should I even—gulp—consider going back to school?

According to psychologist Kathleen Nadeau, director of Chesapeake ADHD Center, the worst jobs for adults with ADHD share two characteristics: they are sedentary and involve prolonged mental concentration.[4] These jobs are long in paperwork and short on opportunities to move around or interact with others; they involve long-term tasks, lots of detail, and a distracting work environment; they are uninteresting, require long hours working alone, and are especially difficult if these characteristics are combined with a boss who is unsympathetic and demanding.

With the inclusion of ADHD as a disability under the Americans with Disabilities Act, employees with ADHD may be eligible for accommodations to help them function more effectively. The basic principle is similar to that involved when kids with ADHD are assisted by a Section 504 accommodation plan in a school system.

> **Key Concept**
>
> With the inclusion of ADHD as a disability under the Americans with Disabilities Act, employees with ADHD may be eligible for accommodations to help them function more effectively.

Even though the idea of job accommodations makes some sense, however, there are some very real problems with its application. First of all, an employee must demonstrate conclusively to his employer that he has ADHD and that his condition interferes seriously with job performance. This means more than just a cursory letter from a doctor, and it also means that a person must admit to problematic job performance.

Second, some individuals who declared their disability to their employers have felt that, as a consequence, they were no longer considered for promotion and may also have been pulled off more desirable jobs.[5] Their declaration, in other words, hurt them more in the long run. These days too, there is no doubt that there is backlash (the national prejudice still exists) against the entire notion of ADHD—especially when many people see the disorder as merely being used as an excuse.

Dr. Nadeau suggests two possible ways of handling the issue of ADHD accommodations on the job. One is to not declare the ADHD unless it is a last resort—either to save a job or to try to buy time if one is close to being fired. The second idea—and perhaps a better and surely less desperate maneuver—is to work out accommodations with one's employer without calling them accommodations and without talking at all about ADHD. If the relationship between employer and employee is good, there are a number of job modifications that might be helpful:

- a private office or less distracting place to work
- working at home
- recording meetings
- more frequent performance appraisals
- getting instructions in writing
- email supervision
- flex time
- extra clerical support

While working with a counselor, adults with ADHD can also take a look at how the work they do might be affected by the use of medication. Most children with ADHD will benefit considerably from stimulants because they have to be in school all day, where they have to sit still and concentrate on material they see as boring. There is more diversity in the lives of adults with ADHD, however, so the uses of stimulant medication are more varied.

An adult diagnosed with ADHD who reviews insurance forms all day, for example, may need to take medication regularly, just as a child in school would. An adult with ADHD who drives a delivery truck for a living, on the other hand, may not need medication at all for that job. Another person with ADHD who does outside sales may not need the meds while driving around the city making calls, but she may need the stimulant medication when Friday afternoon rolls around and it's time to fill out her expense reports. She might also use the medication periodically for recreational reading.

During the process of reevaluating their job situations, many individuals reconsider the possibility of going back to school. Initially, just the thought of school may inspire anxiety—or even downright terror to those with ADHD. However, after experiencing the benefits on concentration that medication often provides, many of these men and women decide to take the plunge. Organizational skills, note taking, reading strategies, and test-taking tactics must be worked on. That old nemesis, homework, must also be attacked aggressively. The good news, however, is that for many adults with ADHD, going back to school—and succeeding—is absolutely thrilling!

The Big Question

We have seen that treatment for adult ADHD exists and can be beneficial. Education about ADHD, medication, counseling, and taking another look at one's job can make life much more satisfying than it ever was before. Self-esteem will rise as a person becomes proud of her accomplishments and develops more satisfying relationships with family, spouse, children, and friends.

Treatment is not perfect though; it involves a lot of work, as well as time and money. Sometimes, it's boring; sometimes, it may seem like it's doing no good. You have to stay in touch with your therapist. Tackling life's big and little jobs that have been chronically avoided, or managing emotions that are persistently exaggerated, requires a lot of elbow grease—day after day. So what's the "big question" about treatment for adult ADHD? As we have discussed, adults with ADHD are good at starting projects but not so good at finishing them. The big question is this: will treatment for ADHD be pursued, or will it simply become one more item on a long list of unfinished endeavors?

For those who have been wrestling with significant ADHD-based impairments for their whole lives, a valid diagnosis of ADHD in adulthood offers several positive—and often revolutionary—benefits. First, a new self-concept: *if I'm not lazy, stupid, or crazy, perhaps I'm hard-working, intelligent, and sane.* Second, greater work effectiveness: increased concentration and organizational skills can make work more interesting and satisfying. Third, better social consciousness: many adults being treated for ADHD find their new abilities to listen and to not interrupt make other people—including family members—much more pleasantly responsive to them. It can be a whole new world!

NOTES

Introduction

1   Walter Roberts, Richard Milich, and Russell A. Barkley, "Primary Symptoms, Diagnostic Criteria, Subtyping, and Prevalence of ADHD," in *Attention-Deficit Hyperactivity Disorder*, ed. Russell A. Barkley (New York: Guilford Press, 2015), 75.

2   G. Polanczyk et al., "The Worldwide Prevalence of ADHD: A Systematic Review and Metaregression Analysis," *The American Journal of Psychiatry* 164 (2007): 942–948.

3   Russell A. Barkley, K. R. Murphy, and M. Fischer, *ADHD in Adults: What the Science Says* (New York: Guilford Press, 2008).

4   George J. DuPaul and Joshua M. Langberg, "Educational Impairments in Children with ADHD," in *Attention-Deficit Hyperactivity Disorder*, ed. Russell A. Barkley (New York: Guilford Press, 2015), 185.

5   Charlotte Johnston and Andrea Chronis-Tuscano, "Families and ADHD," in *Attention-Deficit Hyperactivity Disorder*, ed. Russell A. Barkley (New York: Guilford Press, 2015), 203.

Chapter 1

1   *Diagnostic and Statistical Manual of Mental Disorders: DSM-5* (Washington, DC: American Psychiatric Association, 2013).

2   Ibid.

3   Roberts, Milich, and Barkley, "Primary Symptoms," 66–67.

4   Ibid.

5   Ibid.

6   Virginia Douglas, "Stop, Look, and Listen: The Problem of Sustained Attention and Impulse Control in Hyperactive and Normal Children," *Canadian Journal of Behavioural Science* 4, no. 4 (1972): 259–282.

7   G. J. August et al., "Diagnostic Stability of ADHD in a Community Sample of School-Aged Children Screened for Disruptive Behavior," *Journal of Abnormal Psychology* 26 (1998): 345–356.

8   Russell A. Barkley, "Emotional Dysregulation Is a Core Component of ADHD," in *Attention-Deficit Hyperactivity Disorder*, ed. Russell A. Barkley (New York: Guilford Press, 2015), 81–115.

9   Steven R. Pliszka, "Comorbid Psychiatric Disorders in Children with ADHD," in *Attention-Deficit Hyperactivity Disorder*, ed. Russell A. Barkley (New York: Guilford Press, 2015), 157–158.

10   Ibid.

11   Ibid.

12   Ibid.

13   Elizabeth B. Owens, Stephanie L. Cardoos, and Stephen P. Hinshaw, "Developmental Progression and Gender Differences among Individuals with ADHD," in *Attention-Deficit Hyperactivity Disorder*, ed. Russell A. Barkley (New York: Guilford Press, 2015), 232.

14   Pliszka, "Comorbid Psychiatric Disorders," 141.

15   W. Pelham and M. Bender, "Peer Relationships in Hyperactive Children: Description and Treatment," *Advances in Learning and Behavioral Disabilities* 1 (1982): 365–436.

16   Amori Yee Mikami, "Social Skills Training for Youth with ADHD," in *Attention-Deficit Hyperactivity Disorder*, ed. Russell A. Barkley (New York: Guilford Press, 2015), 569–595.

17   Ibid.

18   Ibid.

19   Russell A. Barkley, *ADHD and the Nature of Self-Control* (New York: Guilford Press, 1997).

20   Edward M. Hallowell and John J. Ratey, *Driven to Distraction: Recognizing and Coping with Attention Deficit Disorder* (New York: Anchor Books, 2011).

Chapter 2

1 Laura E. Berk, *Child Development*, (Pearson, 2013), 646.

2 L. L. Weyandt and B. G. Gudmundsdottir, "Developmental and Neuropsychological Deficits in Children with ADHD," in *Attention-Deficit Hyperactivity Disorder*, ed. Russell A. Barkley (New York: Guilford Press, 2015), 120.

3 Berk, *Child Development*, 461.

4 E. K. Sleator and R. K. Ullmann, "Can the Physician Diagnose Hyperactivity in the Office?" *Pediatrics* 67, no. 1 (1981): 13–17.

5 Russell A. Barkley, *Taking Charge of ADHD: The Complete, Authoritative Guide for Parents* (New York: Guilford Press, 2013).

6 R. Cordier et al., "Comparison of the Play of Children with Attention Deficit Hyperactivity Disorder by Subtypes," *Australian Occupational Therapy Journal* 57, no. 2: 137–145, quoted in Mikami, "Social Skills Training," 573.

Chapter 3

1 Denise Mann, "Study: Fussy Babies Linked to ADHD Risk," WebMD, April 20, 2011, http://www.webmd.com/parenting/baby/news/20110420/study-fussy-babies-linked-to-adhd-risk#1.

2 S. B. Campbell, *Behavior Problems in Preschool Children* (New York: Guilford Press, 1987), quoted in Roberts, Milich, and Barkley, "Primary Symptoms," 60.

3 Russell A. Barkley et al., "The Adolescent Outcome of Hyperactive Children Diagnosed by Research Criteria: III. Mother-Child Interactions, Family Conflicts, and Maternal Psychopathology," *Child Psychology and Psychiatry and Allied Disciplines*: 32, 233–255, quoted in Johnston and Chronis-Tuscano, "Families and ADHD," 200.

4 Weyandt and Gudmundsdottir, "Developmental and Neuropsychological Deficits," 120.

5 Pliszka, "Comorbid Psychiatric Disorders," 141.

6 Ibid.

7 K. M. Kent et al., "The Academic Experience of Male High School Students with ADHD," *Journal of Abnormal Child Psychology* 39, no. 3:

451–462, quoted in DuPaul and Langberg, "Educational Impairments," 175.

8   Gregory A. Fabiano and Nicole K. Schatz, "Driving Risk Interventions for Teens with ADHD," in *Attention-Deficit Hyperactivity Disorder*, ed. Russell A. Barkley (New York: Guilford Press, 2015), 723.

9   Ibid.

10   Roberts, Milich, and Barkley, "Primary Symptoms," 75.

11   T. Kupper et al., "The Negative Impact of Attention-Deficit/Hyperactivity Disorder on Occupational Health in Adults and Adolescents," *International Archives of Occupational and Environmental Health* 85: 837–847, quoted in Barkley, "Educational, Occupational, Dating and Marital, and Financial Impairments in Adults with ADHD," *Attention-Deficit Hyperactivity Disorder*, ed. Russell A. Barkley (New York: Guilford Press, 2015), 326.

12   Russell A. Barkley, "Comorbid Psychiatric Disorders and Psychological Maladjustment in Adults with ADHD," in *Attention-Deficit Hyperactivity Disorder*, ed. Russell A. Barkley (New York: Guilford Press, 2015), 351.

13   Ibid.

Chapter 4

1   Russell A. Barkley, "Etiologies of ADHD," in *Attention-Deficit Hyperactivity Disorder*, ed. Russell A. Barkley (New York: Guilford Press, 2015), 378.

2   Ibid., 358.

3   Ibid.

4   Ibid., 379.

5   Ibid., 378.

6   Ibid., 357.

7   Ibid., 360.

8   Ibid.

9   Ibid., 361.

10   J. B. Schweitzer et al., "Alterations in the Functional Anatomy of Working Memory in Adult Attention Deficit Hyperactivity Disorder," *American Journal of Psychiatry* 157: 278–280, quoted in Barkley, "Etiologies of ADHD," 365; J. M. Swanson, R. D. Baler, and N. D. Volkow, "Understanding the Effects of Stimulant Medications on Cognition in

Individuals with Attention-Deficit Hyperactivity Disorder: A Decade of Progress," *Neuropsychopharmacology* 36, no. 1: 207–226, quoted in Barkley, "Etiologies of ADHD," 368; E. H. Aylward et al., "Basal Ganglia Volumes in Children with Attention-Deficit Hyperactivity Disorder," *Journal of Child Neurology* 11: 112–115, quoted in Barkley, "Etiologies of ADHD," 363.

11   Barkley, "Etiologies of ADHD," 379.

12   Ibid., 369–370.

13   Ibid., 369.

14   Ibid., 378–379.

15   C. K. Connors, *Food Additives and Hyperactive Children* (New York: Plenum Press, 1980), quoted in Russell A. Barkley, "History of ADHD," in *Attention-Deficit Hyperactivity Disorder*, ed. Russell A. Barkley (New York: Guilford Press, 2015), 14.

16   R. Milich, M. Wolraich, and S. Lindgren, "Sugar and Hyperactivity: A Critical Review of Empirical Findings," *Clinical Psychology Review*, no. 6 (1986): 493–513, quoted in Barkley, "History of ADHD," 15.

17   C. S. Hartsough and N. M. Lambert, "Medical Factors in Hyperactive and Normal Children: Prenatal, Developmental, and Health History Findings," *American Journal of Orthopsychiatry*, no. 55 (1985): 190–210, quoted in Russell A. Barkley, "Health Problems and Related Impairments in Children and Adults with ADHD," in *Attention-Deficit Hyperactivity Disorder*, ed. Russell A. Barkley (New York: Guilford Press, 2015), 268.

18   Ibid.

Chapter 5

1   Michael Marmot, *The Status Syndrome: How Social Standing Affects Our Health and Longevity* (New York: Henry Holt and Co., 2005), 12.

2   J. H. Satterfield et al., "A 30-Year Prospective Follow-Up Study of Hyperactive Boys with Conduct Problems: Adult Criminality," *Journal of the American Academy of Child and Adolescent Psychiatry* 46 (2007): 601–610.

3   B. Hoza et al., "Peer-Assessed Outcomes in the Multimodal Treatment Study of Children with Attention Deficit Hyperactivity Disorder," *Journal*

of Clinical Child and Adolescent Psychology 34, no. 1 (2005): 74–86, quoted in Mikami, "Social Skills Training," 572.

4   Roberts, Milich, and Barkley, "Primary Symptoms," 75.

5   Daniel Goleman, *Emotional Intelligence* (New York: Bantam Books, 1995), 36.

6   Ibid.

7   F. S. Kelly et al., "Ability of Schizophrenic Women to Create a Favorable or Unfavorable Impression on an Interviewer," *Journal of Consulting and Clinical Psychology* 36, no. 3 (1971): 404–409.

8   Campbell, *Behavior Problems*, quoted in Roberts, Milich, and Barkley, "Primary Symptoms," 60.

9   *Adult ADHD-Focused Couple Therapy: Clinical Interventions*, ed. Gina Pera and Arthur L. Robin (New York: Routledge, 2016).

10   Barkley, Murphy, and Fischer, *ADHD in Adults*.

Chapter 6

1   Sleator and Ullmann, "Can the Physician Diagnose," 13–17.

2   Campbell, *Behavior Problems,* quoted in Roberts, Milich, and Barkley, "Primary Symptoms," 60.

3   M. Fischer et al., "The Stability of Dimensions of Behavior in ADHD and Normal Children Over an 8-Year Period," *Journal of Abnormal Psychology*, no. 21 (1993): 315–337, quoted in Russell A. Barkley, "Psychological Assessment of Children with ADHD," in *Attention-Deficit Hyperactivity Disorder*, ed. Russell A. Barkley (New York: Guilford Press, 2015), 463.

4   T. M. Achenbach, S. H. McConaughy, and C. T. Howell, "Child/ Adolescent Behavioral and Emotional Problems: Implications of Cross-Informant Correlations for Situational Specificity," *Psychological Bulletin*, no. 101 (1987): 213–232, quoted in Barkley, "Psychological Assessment," 463.

Chapter 7

1   Barkley, "Comorbid Psychiatric Disorders," 351.

2   Pliszka, "Comorbid Psychiatric Disorders," 141.

3   Ibid.

4   Ibid, 152.

5   *DSM-5*, 195.

6   A. Angold and E. J. Costello, "Depressive Comorbidity in Children and Adolescents: Empirical, Theoretical, and Methodological Issues," *American Journal of Psychiatry*, no. 150 (1993): 1779–1791, quoted in Pliszka, "Comorbid Psychiatric Disorders," 151.

7   Ibid., 148.

8   MTA Cooperative Group, "14-Month Randomized Clinical Trial of Treatment Strategies for Children with Attention-Deficit Hyperactivity Disorder," *Archives of General Psychiatry*, no 56. (1999): 1073–1086 (Ibid., 153).

9   A. Rothenberger et al., "Co-Existence of Tic Disorders and Attention-Deficit/Hyperactivity Disorder: Recent Advances in Understanding and Treatment," *European Child and Adolescent Psychiatry* 16, no. 1 (2007), 1–4 (Ibid., 154).

10   Barkley, "Health Problems," 279.

11   P. Corkum et al., "Sleep Disturbances in Children with Attention-Deficit/Hyperactivity Disorder," *Journal of the Academy of Child and Adolescent Psychiatry*, no. 37 (1998): 637–646, quoted in Barkley, "Health Problems," 279.

12   D. F. Connor et al., "Conduct Disorder Subtype and Comorbidity," *Annuls of Clinical Psychiatry* 19, no. 3 (July–September 2007): 161–168.

13   G. J. DuPaul et al., "Comorbidity of LD and ADHD: Implications of *DSM-5* for Assessment and Treatment," *Journal of Learning Disabilities* 46, no. 1 (2013): 43–51.

14   Pliszka, "Comorbid Psychiatric Disorders," 152.

Chapter 8

1   MTA Cooperative Group, "14-Month Randomized Clinical Trial," 1073–1086, quoted in Pliszka, "Comorbid Psychiatric Disorders," 153.

Chapter 9

1   P. C. Kendall and L. Braswell, *Cognitive-Behavioral Therapy for Impulsive Children* (New York: Guilford Press, 1985).

2   V. I. Douglas, "Higher Mental Processes in Hyperactive Children: Implications for Training," in *Treatment of Hyperactive and Learning Disordered Children*, ed. R. Knights and D. Bakker (Baltimore: University Park Press, 1980), 65–92.

3   H. Abikoff, "An Evaluation of Cognitive Behavior Therapy for Hyperactive Children," in *Advances in Clinical Child Psychology*, ed. B. Leahy and A. Kazdin (New York: Plenum Press, 1987), 171–216.

4   M. D. Rapport et al., "Working Memory Deficits in Boys with Attention-Deficit/Hyperactivity Disorder (ADHD): The Contribution of Central Executive and Subsystem Processes," *Journal of Abnormal Child Psychology* 36, no. 6 (2008), in *Attention-Deficit Hyperactivity Disorder*, ed. Russell A. Barkley (New York: Guilford Press, 2015), 664.

5   L. J. Pfiffner, "Social Skills Training," in *Attention-Deficit/Hyperactivity Disorder: Concepts, Controversies, New Directions*, ed. K. McBurnett and L. J. Pfiffner (New York: Informa Healthcare, 2008), 179–190.

6   Barkley, *ADHD and the Nature of Self-Control*, 338–339.

7   G. M. de Voo and P. J. M. Prins, "Social Incompetence in Children with ADHD: Possible Moderators and Mediators in Social-Skills Training," *Clinical Psychology Review*, no. 27 (2007): 1, 78–97.

8   Barkley, *ADHD and the Nature of Self-Control*, 338.

9   Mikami, "Social Skills Training," 569–595.

10 A. M. Chronis, H. A. Jones, and V. L. Raggi, "Evidence-Based Psychosocial Treatments for Children and Adolescents with Attention-Deficit/Hyperactivity Disorder," *Clinical Psychology Review* 26, no. 4 (2006): 486–502.

11 Ibid.

Chapter 10

1   E. Chan, L. A. Rappaport, and K. J. Kemper, "Complementary and Alternative Therapies in Childhood Attention and Hyperactivity Problems," *Journal of Developmental and Behavioral Pediatrics* 24, no. 1 (2003): 4–8.

2   I. Kirsch and G. Sapirstein, "Listening to Prozac but Hearing Placebo: A Meta-Analysis of Antidepressant Medication," *Prevention and Treatment* 1, no. 2 (1998): 1–17.

3   D. A. Wasch Busch et al., "Are There Placebo Effects in the Medication Treatment of Children with Attention-Deficit Hyperactivity Disorder?" *Journal of Developmental Behavioral Pediatrics* 30, no. 2 (2009): 158–168.

4   Amanda Bader and Andrew Adesman, "Complementary and Alternative Medicine for ADHD," in *Attention-Deficit Hyperactivity Disorder*, ed. Russell A. Barkley (New York: Guilford Press, 2015), 729–733.

5   M. R. Leon, "Effects of Caffeine on Cognitive, Psychomotor, and Affective Performance of Children with Attention-Deficit/Hyperactivity Disorder," *Journal of Attention Disorders* 4, no. 1 (2000): 27–47.

6   C. K. Connors et al., "Nicotine Effects on Adults with Attention-Deficit/Hyperactivity Disorder," *Psychopharmacology* 123, no. 1 (1996): 55–63.

7   C. K. Connors, *Food Additives and Hyperactive Children* (New York: Plenum Press, 1980), quoted in Barkley, "History of ADHD," 14.

8   M. H. Bloch and A. Qawasmi, "Omega-3 Fatty Acid Supplementation for the Treatment of Children with Attention-Deficit/Hyperactivity Disorder; Systematic Review and Meta-Analysis," *Journal of the Academy of Child and Adolescent Psychiatry*, no. 50 (2011): 991–1000 in *Attention-Deficit Hyperactivity Disorder*, ed. Russell A. Barkley (New York: Guilford Press, 2015), 639.

9   Ibid, 639; E. J. S. Sonuga-Barke et al., "Nonpharmacological Intervention for ADHD: Systematic Review and Meta-Analyses of Randomized Controlled Trials of Dietary and Psychological Treatments," *American Journal of Psychiatry*, no. 170 (2013): 275–289, in *Attention-Deficit Hyperactivity Disorder*, ed. Russell A. Barkley (New York: Guilford Press, 2015), 640.

10   MTA Cooperative Group, "14-Month Randomized Clinical Trial," 1073–1086, quoted in Pliszka, "Comorbid Psychiatric Disorders," 153.

Chapter 11

1   Barkley, *Taking Charge of ADHD*.

2   "Countertransference," Good Therapy, last modified March 4, 2016, www.goodtherapy.org/blog/psychpedia/countertransference.

3   Anil Chacko et al., "Training Parents of Youth with ADHD," in *Attention-Deficit Hyperactivity Disorder*, ed. Russell A. Barkley (New York: Guilford Press, 2015), 521.

4   American Academy of Pediatrics Committee on Psychosocial Aspects of Child and Family Health, "Guidance for Effective Discipline," *Pediatrics*, no. 101 (1998): 723–728.

5   Johnston and Chronis-Tuscano, "Families and ADHD," 203–204.

6   *DSM-5*, 462.

Chapter 12

1   Daniel F. Connor, "Stimulant and Nonstimulant Medications for Childhood ADHD," in *Attention-Deficit Hyperactivity Disorder*, ed. Russell A. Barkley (New York: Guilford Press, 2015), 666; C. K. Connors, "Forty Years of Methylphenidate Treatment in Attention-Deficit/Hyperactivity Disorder," *Journal of Attention Disorders* 6, no. 1 (2002): 17–30.

2   Connors, "Forty Years of Methylphenidate Treatment," 17–30.

3   Connor, "Stimulant and Nonstimulant Medications," 670.

4   Ibid., 672.

5   P. S. Jensen et al., "3-Year Follow-Up of the NIMH MTA Study," *Journal of the American Academy of Child and Adolescent Psychiatry* 46, no. 8 (2007): 989–1002.

6   Connor, "Stimulant and Nonstimulant Medications," 668.

7   Ibid., 672.

8   Ibid., 673.

9   Barkley, "Health Problems," 298.

10   Y. Tanaka et al., "A Meta-Analysis of the Consistency of Atomoxetine Treatment Effects in Pediatric Patients with Attention-Deficit/ Hyperactivity Disorder from 15 Clinical Trials Across 4 Geographic Regions," *Journal of Child and Adolescent Psychopharmacology* 23, no. 4 (2013): 262–270.

11   R. Jain et al., "Clonidine Extended-Release Tablets for Pediatric Patients with Attention-Deficit/Hyperactivity Disorder," *Journal of the American Academy of Child and Adolescent Psychiatry* 50, no. 2 (2011): 171–179.

12   J. Biederman et al., "A Randomized, Double-Blind, Placebo-Controlled

Study of Guanfacine Extended Release in Children and Adolescents with Attention-Deficit/Hyperactivity Disorder," *Pediatrics* 121, no. 1 (2008): 73–84.

13   J. Biederman et al., "A Comparison of Once Daily and Divided Doses of Modafinil in Children with Attention-Deficit/Hyperactivity Disorder: A Randomized, Double-Blind, and Placebo-Controlled Study," *Journal of Clinical Psychiatry* 67, no. 5 (2006): 727–735.

14   C. K. Connors et al., "Bupropion Hydrochloride in Attention Deficit Disorder with Hyperactivity," *Journal of the American Academy of Child and Adolescent Psychiatry* 35, no. 10 (1996): 1314–1321.

15   J. Biederman and T. J. Spencer, "Psychopharmacological Interventions," *Child and Adolescent Psychiatric Clinics of North America* 17, no. 2 (2008): 439–458.

16   D. F. Connor, K. E. Fletcher, and J. M. Swanson, "A Meta-Analysis of Clonidine for Symptoms of Attention-Deficit/Hyperactivity Disorder," *Journal of the American Academy of Child and Adolescent Psychiatry* 38, no. 12 (1999): 1551–1559.

17   P. B. Chappell et al., "Guanfacine Treatment of Comorbid Attention-Deficit Hyperactivity Disorder and Tourette's Syndrome: Preliminary Clinical Experience," *Journal of the American Academy of Child and Adolescent Psychiatry* 34, no. 9 (1995): 1140–1146.

18   J. Swanson et al., "Evidence, Interpretation, and Qualification from Multiple Reports of Long-Term Outcomes in the Multimodal Treatment Study of Children with ADHD (MTA): Part 1, Executive Summary," *Journal of Attention Disorders* 12, no. 1 (2008): 4–14.

19   B. H. Smith and C. J. Shapiro, "Combined Treatments for ADHD," in *Attention-Deficit Hyperactivity Disorder*, ed. Russell A. Barkley (New York: Guilford Press, 2015), 701.

Chapter 13

1   National Resource Center on ADHD, last modified 2016, www.chadd.org/About-CHADD/National-Resource-Center.aspx.

2   Education for All Handicapped Children Act of 1975, 20 U.S.C. § 1401 (1975).

3   Individuals with Disabilities Education Act, 20 U.S.C. § 1400 (1990).

4   Individuals with Disabilities Education Improvement Act of 2004, 20 U.S.C. § 1400 (2004).

5   Rehabilitation Act of 1973, 29 U.S.C. § 701 (1973).

6   Individuals with Disabilities Education Improvement Act of 2004, 20 U.S.C. § 1400 (2004); Rehabilitation Act of 1973, 29 U.S.C. § 701 (1973).

7   Individuals with Disabilities Education Improvement Act of 2004, 20 U.S.C. § 1400 (2004).

8   Individuals with Disabilities Education Improvement Act of 2004, 20 U.S.C. § 1400 (2004); Rehabilitation Act of 1973, 29 U.S.C. § 701 (1973).

9   *DSM-5.*

10 "Documentation Requirements," Division of Disability Resources and Educational Services, University of Illinois at Champaign-Urbana, accessed August 27, 2016, http://disability.illinois.edu/applying-services/documentation-requirements.

11 R. B. Eiraldi, J. A. Mautone, and T. J. Power, "Strategies for Implementing Evidence-Based Psychosocial Interventions for Children with Attention-Deficit/Hyperactivity Disorder," *Child and Adolescent Psychiatric Clinics of North America*, no. 21 (2012): 145–159.

Chapter 14

1   *DSM-5*, 61.

2   Barkley, *Taking Charge of ADHD*.

Chapter 15

1   Roberts, Milich, and Barkley, "Primary Symptoms," 75.

2   Barkley, "Comorbid Psychiatric Disorders," 351.

3   J. T. Nigg, "Attention-Deficit/Hyperactivity Disorder and Adverse Health Outcomes," *Clinical Psychology Review*, no. 33 (2013): 215–228.

4   Ibid.

5   Ibid.

6   T. Vaa, "ADHD and Relative Risk of Accidents in Road Traffic: A Meta-Analysis," *Accident Analysis and Prevention*, no. 62 (2014), 415–425.

7   Barkley, Murphy, and Fischer, *ADHD in Adults*.

8   G. B. DeQuiros and M. Kinsbourne, "Adult ADHD: Analysis of Self-Ratings on a Behavior Questionnaire," *Annals of the New York Academy of Sciences*, no. 931 (2001): 140–147.

9   K. R. Murphy and Russell A. Barkley, "Attention-Deficit Hyperactivity Disorder in Adults: Comorbidity and Adaptive Impairments," *Comprehensive Psychiatry*, no. 37 (1996): 393–401.

10   Ibid.

11   Ibid.

12   J. Biederman et al., "Patterns of Psychiatric Comorbidity, Cognition, and Psychosocial Functioning in Adults with Attention-Deficit Hyperactivity Disorder," *American Journal of Psychiatry*, no. 150 (1993): 1792–1798.

13   Pliszka, "Comorbid Psychiatric Disorders," 141.

Chapter 16

1   Roberts, Milich, and Barkley, "Primary Symptoms," 75.

2   *DSM-5*, 59–60.

3   Stephen B. McCarney and Tamara J. Arthaud, *Attention Deficit Disorder Evaluation Scale* (Columbia: Hawthorne Educational Services, 2013).

4   Sleator and Ullmann, "Can the Physician Diagnose," 13–17.

Chapter 17

1   K. Kelly and P. Ramundo, *You Mean I'm Not Lazy, Stupid, or Crazy?* (New York: Scribner, 2006).

2   J. B. Prince et al., "Pharmacotherapy of ADHD in Adults," in *Attention-Deficit Hyperactivity Disorder*, ed. Russell A. Barkley (New York: Guilford Press, 2015), 826.

3   Ibid., 847–850.

4   Kathleen Nadeau, *ADD in the Workplace: Choices, Changes, and Challenges* (New York: Routledge, 1997), 6.

5   Ibid., 203–214.

SELECT BIBLIOGRAPHY

American Psychiatric Association. *Diagnostic and Statistical Manual of Mental Disorders: DSM-5.* Washington, DC: American Psychiatric Association, 2013.

August, G. J. et al. "Diagnostic Stability of ADHD in a Community Sample of School-Aged Children Screened for Disruptive Behavior." *Journal of Abnormal Psychology* 26 (1998): 345–356.

Barkley, Russell A. *ADHD and the Nature of Self-Control.* New York: Guilford Press, 1997.

———, K. R. Murphy, and M. Fischer. *ADHD in Adults: What the Science Says.* New York: Guilford Press, 2008.

———, ed. *Attention-Deficit Hyperactivity Disorder.* New York: Guilford Press, 2015.

———. "Comorbid Psychiatric Disorders and Psychological Maladjustment in Adults with ADHD." In Barkley, *Attention-Deficit Hyperactivity Disorder,* 343–355.

———. "Educational, Occupational, Dating and Marital, and Financial Impairments in Adults with ADHD." In Barkley, *Attention-Deficit Hyperactivity Disorder,* 314–342.

———. "Emotional Dysregulation Is a Core Component of ADHD." In Barkley, *Attention-Deficit Hyperactivity Disorder,* 81–115.

———. "Etiologies of ADHD." In Barkley, *Attention-Deficit Hyperactivity Disorder,* 356–390.

————. "Health Problems and Related Impairments in Children and Adults with ADHD." In Barkley, *Attention-Deficit Hyperactivity Disorder*, 267–313.

————. "History of ADHD." In Barkley, *Attention-Deficit Hyperactivity Disorder*, 3–50.

————. "Psychological Assessment of Children with ADHD." In Barkley, *Attention-Deficit Hyperactivity Disorder*, 455–474.

————. *Taking Charge of ADHD: The Complete, Authoritative Guide for Parents*. New York: Guilford Press, 2013.

Berk, Laura E. *Child Development*. Pearson, 2013.

Biederman, J., and T. J. Spencer. "Psychopharmacological Interventions." *Child and Adolescent Psychiatric Clinics of North America* 17, no. 2 (2008): 439–458.

Chacko, Anil et al. "Training Parents of Youth with ADHD." In Barkley, *Attention-Deficit Hyperactivity Disorder*, 513–536.

Connor, Daniel F. "Stimulant and Nonstimulant Medications for Childhood ADHD." In Barkley, *Attention-Deficit Hyperactivity Disorder*, 666–685.

Douglas, Virginia. "Stop, Look, and Listen: The Problem of Sustained Attention and Impulse Control in Hyperactive and Normal Children." *Canadian Journal of Behavioural Science* 4, no. 4 (1972): 259–282.

DuPaul, George J. et al. "Comorbidity of LD and ADHD: Implications of *DSM-5* for Assessment and Treatment." *Journal of Learning Disabilities* 46, no. 1 (2013): 43–51.

————, and Joshua M. Langberg. "Educational Impairments in Children with ADHD." In Barkley, *Attention-Deficit Hyperactivity Disorder*, 169–190.

Fabiano, Gregory A., and Nicole K. Schatz. "Driving Risk Interventions for Teens with ADHD." In Barkley, *Attention-Deficit Hyperactivity Disorder*, 705–727.

Goleman, Daniel. *Emotional Intelligence*. New York: Bantam Books, 1995.

Hallowell, Edward M., and John J. Ratey. *Driven to Distraction: Recognizing and Coping with Attention Deficit Disorder*. New York: Anchor Books, 2011.

Johnston, Charlotte, and Andrea Chronis-Tuscano. "Families and ADHD." In Barkley, *Attention-Deficit Hyperactivity Disorder*, 191–209.

Kelly, F. S. et al. "Ability of Schizophrenic Women to Create a Favorable or Unfavorable Impression on an Interviewer." *Journal of Consulting and Clinical Psychology* 36, no. 3 (1971): 404–409.

Kelly, K. and P. Ramundo. *You Mean I'm Not Lazy, Stupid, or Crazy?* New York: Scribner, 2006.

Kendall, P. C., and L. Braswell. *Cognitive-Behavioral Therapy for Impulsive Children*. New York: Guilford Press, 1985.

Mann, Denise. "Study: Fussy Babies Linked to ADHD Risk." WebMD. April 20, 2011. http://www.webmd.com/parenting/baby/news/20110420/study-fussy-babies-linked-to-adhd-risk#1.

Marmot, Michael. *The Status Syndrome: How Social Standing Affects Our Health and Longevity*. New York: Henry Holt & Co., 2005.

McBurnett, K., and L. J. Pfiffner, ed. *Attention-Deficit/Hyperactivity Disorder: Concepts, Controversies, New Directions*. New York: Informa Healthcare, 2008.

McCarney, Stephen B., and Tamara J. Arthaud. *Attention Deficit Disorder Evaluation Scale*. Columbia: Hawthorne Educational Services, 2013.

Mikami, Amori Yee. "Social Skills Training for Youth with ADHD." In Barkley, *Attention-Deficit Hyperactivity Disorder*, 569–595.

Nadeau, Kathleen. *ADD in the Workplace: Choices, Changes, and Challenges*. New York: Routledge, 1997.

Owens, Elizabeth B., Stephanie L. Cardoos, and Stephen P. Hinshaw. "Developmental Progression and Gender Differences among Individuals with ADHD." In Barkley, *Attention-Deficit Hyperactivity Disorder*, 223–255.

Pelham, W., and M. Bender. "Peer Relationships in Hyperactive Children: Description and Treatment." *Advances in Learning and Behavioral Disabilities* 1(1982): 365–436.

Pera, Gina, and Arthur L Robin, ed. *Adult ADHD-Focused Couple Therapy: Clinical Interventions*. New York: Routledge, 2016.

Pliszka, Steven R. "Comorbid Psychiatric Disorders in Children with ADHD." In Barkley, *Attention-Deficit Hyperactivity Disorder*, 140–168.

Polanczyk, G, et al. "The Worldwide Prevalence of ADHD: A Systematic Review and Metaregression Analysis." *The American Journal of Psychiatry* 164 (2007): 942–948.

Roberts, Walter, Richard Milich, and Russell A. Barkley. "Primary Symptoms, Diagnostic Criteria, Subtyping, and Prevalence of ADHD." In Barkley, *Attention-Deficit Hyperactivity Disorder*, 51–80.

Satterfield, J. H. et al. "A 30-Year Prospective Follow-Up Study of Hyperactive Boys with Conduct Problems: Adult Criminality." *Journal of the American Academy of Child and Adolescent Psychiatry* 46 (2007): 601–610.

Sleator, E. K., and R. K. Ullman. "Can the Physician Diagnose Hyperactivity in the Office?" *Pediatrics* 67, no. 1 (1981): 13–17.

Weyandt, L. L., and B. G. Gudmundsdottir. "Developmental and Neuropsychological Deficits in Children with ADHD." In Barkley, *Attention-Deficit Hyperactivity Disorder*, 116–139.

INDEX

D

M

ABOUT THE AUTHOR

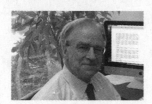 **DR. THOMAS W. PHELAN** is an internationally renowned expert, author, and lecturer on child discipline and attention-deficit/hyperactivity disorder. A registered PhD clinical psychologist, he appears frequently on radio and TV. Dr. Phelan practices and works in the western suburbs of Chicago.

IF YOU ENJOYED *ALL ABOUT ADHD...*

check out these other products from
Thomas W. Phelan, PhD

Did You Know? *1-2-3 Magic*, *1-2-3 Magic for Kids*, and the *1-2-3 Magic* DVDs are also available in Spanish!

1-2-3 Magic
Effective Discipline for Children 2–12

1-2-3 Magic DVD
Managing Difficult Behavior in Children 2–12

More 1-2-3 Magic DVD
Encouraging Good Behavior, Independence, and Self-Esteem

1-2-3 Magic Workbook
A user-friendly, illustrated companion to the *1-2-3 Magic* book that includes case studies, self-evaluation questions, and exercises

1-2-3 Magic in the Classroom
Effective Discipline for Pre-K through Grade 8

1-2-3 Magic for Teachers DVD
Effective Classroom Discipline Pre-K through Grade 8

1-2-3 Magic for Kids
Helping Your Children Understand the New Rules

1-2-3 Magic for Christian Parents
Effective Discipline for Children 2–12

1-2-3 Magic Starter Kit
Accessories to help you get started with the 1-2-3 Magic program

Tantrums! Book and DVD
Managing Meltdowns in Public and Private

Surviving Your Adolescents
The Dos and Don'ts of Managing Life with Teens

Visit www.123magic.com